AN OUNCE OF PREVENTION

IS WORTH MORE THAN YOU CAN IMAGINE

ALLEN DAUGHERTY

An Ounce of Prevention
Is Worth More Than You Can ImagineAllen Daugherty

Contents

Introduction..1
Preface..5

Chapter 1.   Conscious Awareness vs Autopilot...................7
Chapter 2.   Safety Takes Time, But It's Worth It! 13
Chapter 3.   Take Safety Seriously....................................19
Chapter 4.   Learn From Close Calls.................................24
Chapter 5.   Novice, Confident, Dangerous......................29
Chapter 6.   Don't Ignore the Warnings 34
Chapter 7.   Safety for Infants and Small Children............41
Chapter 8.   Raising Safety Conscious Children.................49
Chapter 9.   Danger! Danger! We Have a Teenager 53
Chapter 10. Adult Safety..59
Chapter 11. Safety at Home..63
Chapter 12. Automobile Safety..71
Chapter 13. Enduring Illness or Enjoying Wellness............80
Chapter 14. What You Are Eating May Be Eating You!......83
Chapter 15. Exercise 87
Chapter 16. Preventive Healthcare and Screenings.............91
Chapter 17. Procrastination: Prevention and Safety Can't
             Wait! 98
Chapter 18. An Ounce of Tips.......................................102

Conclusion..107
Appendix 1...109
Statistics 113

Introduction

I am so glad you are reading this book. Hopefully, as you read it, the value of prevention will become clearer than ever before. My name is Allen Daugherty, and I am the founder of P.H.A.S.E., Preventive Healthcare and Safety Engagement. The mission of the P.H.A.S.E. team is to help people avoid accidents and illnesses that can devastate and, even worse, end their lives.

We want our message to help you understand the importance of prevention and how it can impact your life. I am sure you have heard of defensive driving? Well, we call this "defensive living." We are a brand-new organization, but I am sure it won't be long before we have testimonials on our website from people telling us how engaging prevention has helped them to avert an undesirable event, accident, or developing a severe medical condition. There are many other organizations like ours and I recommend you visit their sites for even more information.

Hopefully by the time you have finished reading, you and your family will have elevated the importance of prevention in your lives. You can then help others by referring this book, our website, or just sharing some of the things that stuck out to you. As we look at examples, many of you will shake your head and say, *"Wow, I never thought of it like that."* Please pass that on to others so that they too can learn the valuable lesson that small preventive practices can prevent a lifetime of misery or worse...

I will refer to a couple of my other books which go into more detail on some of the subjects we are going to discuss. I write in a very simple, conversational manner so please don't expect a lot of big, technical words—mainly because I don't know many—and be prepared for a little humor along the way. We are dealing with a very serious subject but a smile once in a while helps with the reading.

I kid you not, one year I was on Hunting Island, South Carolina, fishing. I ran across the sand along one of the lagoons in my bare feet to catch up with my son. I split my heel wide open on an oyster shell leaving a nice, long trail of blood along the shore.

The very next year, I was working on my roof. (You guessed already?) I had a ladder on top of the porch roof working on the top roof. The fine wood fibers from the rotten wood had made the porch roof slightly slippery. I was on the ladder, pounding shingles on the top roof, when the ladder started to slip. It fell, bringing me along with it and I hit the porch roof, slid off, and fell to the ground. My left ankle was at a ninety-degree angle—the wrong way.

The following year, (yep... still not kidding), I was in a hurry to get the grass cut. It was wet and I was backing up with a push mower and—you are so smart, got it right again—I slipped and pulled the lawnmower up on my foot. I now only have nine and one quarter toes left. I know what you are saying, *"Boy, the irony of this guy writing a book about safety."* But if I share these things with you, then you will be more careful, right? Well, that's the ticket!

After the three accidents, I remember saying, *"Boy, if I only would have..."* or Boy if I only hadn't..." So therefore, this book is dedicated to all of us who have said that, and its purpose is to keep us and others from making similar mistakes.

Ever think about the game, Russian Roulette? Can you imagine putting a bullet in a revolver and spinning the barrel leaving you with no idea where that bullet was, putting the gun to your head, and pulling the trigger? It's only a one-out- of-six chance that the gun will fire. But do you really want to play those odds with your life? How about your children's lives? Yet, many of the things we do tend to add bullets, which increases the risk. I know it sounds ludicrous but that is what we are actually doing.

I guarantee that even though you may not see many new ideas in this book, you will soon realize how important it is to seriously focus on the things you already do know about preventive healthcare and safety.

Preface

As you begin your journey through this book, I want you to notice how very serious and complicated things can be broken down into very simple concepts. We are going to be talking about various preventive health and safety topics, but the book is designed to get you to think about just a few elementary things.

1. Every day, unfortunately, just normal, routine life presents risks. **QUESTION:** *Is what you are doing or not doing increasing or decreasing those risks?* For example, putting your seatbelt on is decreasing the risk; failing to undergo routine health screening is increasing the risk. This theme will be threaded throughout the book.
2. We will mention the '*stop, pause, and think*' phrase many times. You can probably imagine what the 'stop' and 'think' represents, but what about the 'pause'? This is a crucial addition.
3. Looking down the road at what could happen will often help us exercise preventive measures when we do things. Do you really want to spend the rest of your life living with the thought that the tragedy which occurred could and should have been prevented?
4. Always comparing the ounce of prevention with the worst-case scenario will guide you into doing the right

thing. (i.e., Checking the smoke detectors vs having your house burn down at night while you and your family are asleep).

5. Remember; *An Ounce of Prevention* is (always) worth more than you can imagine!

Chapter 1

Conscious Awareness vs Autopilot

What controls the things you do and how you do them? Your mind, very good. (I heard a guy say one time, "My wife". Only one honest man in the whole crowd). For our purposes, let's divide our mind into two sections: the conscious mind and the subconscious mind. The *conscious mind* allows our actions to be done deliberately after thought and consideration. The *subconscious mind* controls the things we do automatically without really having to think about them. I call this the 'autopilot'.

I have written a book that elaborates this very well, *Reincarnate Now*, but I want to explain it briefly here. I do not have to deliberately think about brushing my teeth every time I brush my teeth. It is just a habit I have developed, and I do it automatically without thinking about it or making any decisions. I set my alarm every night; its automatic. I take my medications every morning; its automatic. I take a shower every Saturday night; it's… (Ha ha! I just wanted to see if you were still with me…).

The things we just talked about, and many others, are great things to have on autopilot. (Better known as *habits*). The more, good things we do automatically, the less chance there is that they will be missed. For example: I take all my medications in the morning. A while back, I was prescribed a medication which I was supposed to take after my evening meal. I did it the first night, missed one, then hit two then missed two. To make a long story short, I had to set a reminder to take that pill until it became routine. Once I had it on autopilot, I never missed it again.

Unfortunately, we have some things on autopilot that shouldn't be. I would have to describe my dietary habits as 'grazing.' I just go from place-to-place nibbling on whatever I can find. I don't decide to do it, I just do it. *'Now, should I get a chip out of that bag and eat it?'* I am trying to lose weight, my cholesterol is high, and I am supposed to watch my sodium; so, I should probably pass on it. Do I do that? Nope. It's grab, open, in, chew, and gone.

Do smokers say, *'OK, that was a great meal. Do I want to go out now and smoke a cigarette?'* Not really, they just do it. I have heard people slip and cuss during important meetings. They didn't think about it, it was just automatic. How many things do you do that are on autopilot? Keep adding the positive things and try to eliminate the bad habits. So, what on earth does all that have to do with safety and preventive healthcare? Since we do so many things subconsciously, meaning we really don't think about what we are doing, we don't think about danger or prevention either.

The illustrations I will be using are made up—unless I say they really happened. Events very similar to these examples do happen to people all the time, just like this one below…

A mother is out in the front yard with her three-year-old who was playing in a sandbox. She suddenly heard her cell phone ring in the house; so she jumped up, and ran into the house to get it. Now, there is a country road at the end of the yard, about thirty feet from where the little boy was playing. It is not a real busy road, but there is some traffic.

Don't shudder yet, I think this one will have a happy ending. When she came back outside, she noticed that her son was up, walking around and guess what? Yes indeed, a car was coming. Thankfully it was being driven by a sixty- five-year-old bald guy who always slows down when he sees children. (Hey, that's me.) But let's replay that scenario. This time, Mom gets up, she stops, pauses, and thinks (which she did NOT do before). *"I can't leave him out here so close to the road. He is quick and may run out in front of a car."* So, she takes him with her into the house to get her phone. But you say, what if she misses the call? I am so glad that I have been advising people for so many years. It makes me eminently qualified to give very educated answers to perplexing questions like this. *"She can call them back"*. If you don't get anything else out of this book, please memorize this very important sequence, *stop, pause, and think.*

So, what exactly is the pause? In the first scenario, she heard the phone ring, stopped for a second and thought. *"I left my phone in the house."* She then got up and ran in. In the second scenario, she did the same thing, but this time she PAUSED for a minute to really evaluate the situation and then thought, *"I can't leave him out here so close to the road."* The pause gave her the time to weigh the prevention against what possibly could happen; and she made the right choice.

Always weigh the worst-case scenarios for both the prevention and the risk, and one hundred percent of the time, the prevention will be worth it. I could miss the call (using prevention), or my son could be struck by a car on the road, (risk). No brainer, right? That is why we need that *pause*; to think it out entirely and realistically.

We rush through life so quickly that we hate stopping for anything. Mark this down and remember it; *rushing decreases the likelihood of employing preventive practices and thus increases the risk of adverse events.* I wish I had a nickel for every time I heard someone say, *"I was just in such a hurry that…"* or *"I just really didn't have the time to…"*

I mentioned earlier that I also talk a lot about one of my favorite terms, *'Conscious Awareness'.* Rushing through life also makes us rely on autopilot a bit more and thus, we are not continually consciously aware of our immediate circumstances. Just like cutting the wet grass that day. I was in a hurry, and I wanted to get that grass cut so I was going full speed. I should have stopped, paused and thought, *'I have slipped many times on wet grass before. If I do it while I'm cutting the grass, my foot could slide under that lawn mower, HMMMM. I guess I should either wait until the grass dries a bit more, (best choice), or cut very slowly and be extra careful.'* But I didn't pause long enough to weigh the risk, so the left side of the sock on my right foot is a bit loose.

Now, I am going to play with you a bit… First, here is another fact. We talked about things which we do subconsciously, and we talked about rushing and how both of those things decrease the changes of us employing many preventive practices. It is even more of a problem when we rush doing the things that we do subconsciously, (combining the two).

When I iron my shirts, I automatically unplug the iron after the last sleeve. (I do the sleeves last, don't you? No, I have never stopped, paused, or thought about it—smarty pants). Anyhow, sometimes, I must think back and ask myself, *'Did I unplug the iron?'* See, I do it so routinely, it leaves very little memory, particularly when I am rushing. Now have you ever stopped and wondered, *"Did I unplug the iron?" "Did I lock the door?" "Did I turn the thermostat back up?" "Did I turn my headlights off??"* It happens all the time and some of those things are benign, but it can take a disastrous twist.

I am a positive person and hate talking about bad things but since this book is on prevention, on occasion, I will have to. To illustrate this point, I am sure you have heard about parents who have left children in the back seat of their car, and worked all day, only to return to a horrifying scene. Taking the child to day care and driving to work were both autopilot functions and rushing may have caused them to forget the first step. *What a nightmare!* Slow down, keep tragedies like that from happening. How many times have you heard the phrase, *"Well, I just didn't stop to think"?* Don't become another person who regretfully says it. Slow down and be more consciously aware of how you can prevent catastrophes, not be a part of them.

Now what about preventive healthcare? I hear all the time, *"Well, my feeling is, if it ain't broke, don't fix it. I haven't been to the doctor, dentist, or even had an eye exam in years. If I need to someday, I'll go."* More people have that attitude than you think, and it is one of the reasons I formed P.H.A.S.E. and am writing this book. I hate to say it, but you are adding bullets to your Russian roulette game. I doubt that if you are reading this book, you hold to that belief, but if you do, please keep reading.

I have been working in Dialysis for over twenty-eight years. Dialysis is for people whose kidneys quit functioning. They either have to dialyze at home, (best option), almost every day or they have to go into a dialysis center three days a week to get a dialysis treatment. If they don't, well, without getting a transplant, they will die.

It is a very sad condition, and without getting a kidney transplant, they must stay on dialysis for the rest of their lives.

The even sadder fact is that thousands of patients who are on dialysis could have prevented their kidney failure. The two main causes of kidney failure are high blood pressure and diabetes. If diagnosed early enough and treated properly, patients can avert, or at least delay, any resulting kidney failure.

Due to the recent developments in cancer treatments, the survival rate for cancer patients has increased tremendously, *if diagnosed early.* Routine screenings at recommended timeframes have saved thousands of lives. So, why don't people take advantage of them? Because they do not stop, pause, and think about the consequences. They just brush it off, it's automatic, no decision-making involved, and since we have created such hectic lifestyles, we just don't take the time.

Now, our subconscious mind can be trained to include some preventive measures—I bet you do some of them. When I get in the car, I automatically put my seatbelt on. No thinking needed; I just do it. (Plus, I hate that annoying *ding, ding,* if I don't). When I weed eat, I automatically put my safety glasses on. When it is time for an appointment or a screening, I don't have to think about it, I just get the appointment made. (I haven't always been that way. Quadruple bypasses teach you a bit).

It takes some time and persistence to make good things and habits a part of your subconscious routine. If you don't believe me, start a diet or exercise program. It starts with doing it, doing it all the time, and continuously doing it until it becomes a habit. Examine that autopilot frequently and work hard to get the good in and the bad out. You will be amazed how many battles in life you will overcome.

Chapter 2

Safety Takes Time, But It's Worth It!

Yes, we are going to talk some more about rushing. I'll try to hurry—get it? Rushing... *try to hurry.* I know, I know, the humor just rolls out). The best way to demonstrate this point is to introduce you to a few people who learned the lesson about rushing, the hard way. Now, I am making these scenarios up, but I assure you, they happen all the time. Again, that is the purpose of this book. I am hoping that all of you will really take to heart what I am saying so you can prevent and, not experience, any terrible events.

Here is Bob. Bob is a good son and likes to help his aging father with his yard work. His dad can ride the mower pretty well, but there are some areas that need cutting with a push mower and then the ever-fun weed eating—I hate weed eating. One Saturday, Bob got a call from some of his friends; they wanted him to go golfing later that afternoon. He remembered telling his dad he would go over that day and do the weed eating for him. If he *HURRIED*, he could get it done and still make his golf outing.

He was about halfway to his dad's house when he realized he had forgotten his safety goggles. If he turned around to get them, he would be late meeting the guys at the golf course. He started thinking, *"I will be really careful; it will be OK. Besides, I don't ever remember taking a hit on the safety glasses. The weed eater shoots most of the stuff straight out. I haven't been golfing in a while and I don't want to miss our tee time."*

We will end the story right there. You are asking, *"Well, what happened?"*—you see, that question in itself brings up a huge point, so thanks for reminding me. When we do not think about or take the time to be safe, it leads us to *Potential Danger.* Potential danger, then, utilizes *Chance* to determine the outcome. It may not cause any harm at all, or it could produce a terrible outcome.

That brings us to my next question; *"Are you a gambler, you know, like our Russian Roulette game?"*... *"Well, no, I never even buy a lottery ticket."* The truth is any lack of prevention you exhibit leads to potential danger and after that; you are gambling. It may turn out OK; it may not, but you are rolling the dice. Remember the title of the book? What... you forgot already? An *Ounce of Prevention is Worth More Than You Can Imagine.* (Had to look myself, Ha ha!).

When you buy a twenty-dollar lottery ticket, what are you risking? You are risking the twenty-dollars. If you win, you may get much more BUT if you lose, there goes your twenty-dollar. So, what was Bob risking? Loss of sight in one, or perhaps even, both eyes. Working backwards a bit, how do you keep from encountering this risk? By not leaving things up to chance. And how do you keep from leaving things up to chance? By avoiding potential danger. And how do you do that? **PREVENTION**. And you will be more likely to use prevention when you stop, *PAUSE*, and thought about it.

Since this is one of our first examples, let's run with it a little. Here is our nice guy Bob, sitting in the Emergency Room after learning that he permanently lost sight in his right eye. *What a tragedy.* Now, if he had really PAUSED and thought about, he could have come up with several options. He could have called ahead and asked his dad if he had some goggles or if he could do some weed eating that morning and the rest later so he could make his golf outing. Then all would have been well—I bet you can think of more options as well. Don't rush or make a quick decision using a distracted mind. (Think about that first golf swing). Take your time to be safe.

Now, I do have to throw in a disclaimer here: sometimes bad things happen even though you do all you can, but you still can't prevent them. People who don't drink or smoke still get cancer. Even the most careful drivers still get into accidents. You can do everything right, and still get hurt. Prevention does not eliminate the risk, but it does lower it. Think of a see-saw. When the prevention goes up on one side, the risk goes down on the other. But remember, the opposite is also true. Very little prevention creates a lot more risk.

Nancy is a very careful driver. She gets into her car, adjusts the mirrors, puts her seatbelt on, and starts on her journey. Both hands are on the wheel, the radio isn't blaring, she ignores a couple of text messages, follows all the laws of the road, and practices very safe driving.

She is doing everything to prevent getting into an accident. You can almost guess what I am going to say next, right? A car is coming from the other direction, you can tell he is a bit pre-occupied with something else besides driving. Just at the wrong time, he swerves over into Nancy's lane and an accident occurs. Did Nancy do everything she could to prevent an accident? Yes, she did, but sometimes they still happen.

But think of this. If 1,000 Nancy's were driving and 1,000 drivers like the other guy were driving, which group do you think would experience more accidents? Correct, the other driver. So, that means that their risk of being in an accident is greater because they did not work to prevent it. *You cannot totally eradicate the risk of being involved in an accident, but you sure can decrease it.*

Let's see what Leslie is up to. She is nineteen years old and babysitting her five-year-old little brother. They always have cookies and milk in the afternoon while they watch his favorite TV show but, on this particular day, they were out of milk.

"Leslie, I want milk and cookies."

"I know, but we don't have any milk."

"We can go to the store." (I don't know about you, but I am betting on this kid).

"Oh, I suppose. Oh no wait, I just remembered, your car seat is in Mom's car. She forgot to leave it. She'll be home in an hour."

"Please Leslie." (She is toast now). "I want milk and cookies."

"Well, OK, I guess it's not far and we will be really careful."

Do you want to guess how many children are killed each year because they were either not restrained or not in an appropriate seat for their age? Yes, it was only five miles to the store. Do you also know that a great majority of accidents happen within five miles of home? Since this is a made-up story, I don't have to continue with what happened. I think we know what could have happened. By the way, was it worth taking a chance like that for an hour? (I'll let you answer that one, I think you are smart enough…).

Chuck needs to change a lightbulb in a ceiling light fixture. He hates that fixture because it is hard to maneuver. It has been out for a while, and he was increasing his risk of being injured by his wife. (Ha ha, prevention guys). He forgot he had left the step ladder out in the garage and was a bit perturbed that he was going to have to go get it. To save time—oh no—he grabbed a kitchen chair, stood on it, and started working on the light. Wonder how long a construction worker would be out with a broken right arm? Let's ask Chuck. Chapter 1: Stop, pause, and think. Chapter 2: Take the time to be safe... See how it all comes together?

Fred was so happy. He bought his wife a new recliner for her birthday and his son was coming over to help him unload it. He wanted it in the living room before his wife got home, but his son called stating that he was going to be late. Now, it was going to be close timing. Fred decided to try and get the couch in by himself. He carefully backed his truck up to the porch and was able to get the recliner out of the truck and onto the porch. The recliner was too wide to slide through the door, so Fred had to turn it on its side and open it up to get it through. As he did, he heard a noise. No, the recliner was fine, but Fred couldn't move... his back was out. Now, was that a safe act? No. Why did he do it? Because he was in a hurry. He didn't employ any safety prevention measures, entered into potential danger, and took a chance. So many times, when you see something like that, you will hear, *"I should have..."* Yes, Fred, you should have just waited.

John is a truck driver. In his twenties and thirties, he had a good exercise routine and watched what he ate. He started accepting longer and overnight drives, and soon both the diet and exercise plan went out the window. He began to gain weight slowly and steadily through his forties and fifties. He noticed he had much less energy and was having some trouble breathing when he exerted himself. Friends and family tried to talk John into getting a physical exam, but he said he was fine and didn't have time. *"Just a few more rides and I can hang this up and then I'll get a physical."* Well, he had his few more rides: one in an ambulance and two in a hearse. You say, you are really trying to scare me—well perhaps, but how about this for scary? Over 800,000 people die each year in the US from heart disease. That accounts for about a third of the deaths, and by the way, heart disease is still the leading cause of death. Don't gamble with your life, take prevention seriously.

Time is the ounce. Be willing to take the time to be safe. These were some made up examples, but I assure you, everyday people get seriously injured and/or killed by not taking the time to be safe. Others fail to use preventive healthcare and become terminally ill or die. Don't be a statistic in my next book.

Chapter 3

Take Safety Seriously

The phrase, *"Ah, it could never happen to me"* has, in many cases, become someone's last words. Safety and health must be taken seriously and thus prevention as well. The reason why people do not take it seriously is because they do not stop, pause, and take the time to think and consider what is at risk.

Phil and Willie are checking out the electrical layout on a construction site. Phil grabs two hard hats and attempts to hand one to Willie.

Willie said, "Nah, we are only going to be here a few minutes." He said that just as they walked past a sign that said, 'HARD HAT AREA; Hard Hats Required to Proceed Past This Point.'

It's amazing how stubborn we can be at times. Just put the hard hat on Willie... I mean, what is at risk? Well, if a hard object fell through the site from several floors above, it could be a broken neck and total paralysis, a broken back, but most likely, a lethal head injury and a body bag. Back in the old days, (in a coal mine far, far away... sorry, got carried away), coal mines, steel mills, construction sites, and other workplaces were very unsafe. Many years later, safety engineers observed the worksites and instituted safety measures which have saved thousands of lives and serious injuries. But they only work if they are followed.

Again, people never even consider that they could be the ones involved. *"I won't fall off the roof,"* (I personally don't say that one anymore), *"I won't get in a wreck, nothing is going to fall on me," "I'm not going to get hit in the eye; it just won't happen to me." "I feel fine, there is no cancer in my family. Mammograms hurt and besides, I check myself." "I forgot the sunscreen but that's OK, I want a real dark tan. I'll be fine."*

If you want to start a very sad hobby, contact those who have had serious injuries. Get the story as to why they are now blind, or why they are paralyzed, or what happened to their arm, or why they can't walk anymore. Those conditions are sad enough but many of them are even sadder when you think about how easily the accident which caused the condition could have been avoided. Then talk to those who developed serious medical conditions because they resisted any type of preventive health measures. Imaging lying on your death bed with cancer or another terminal disease thinking back to all the opportunities you had to go for screenings.

I can't imagine going through life blind especially knowing my disregard for safety caused me to be that way. How about having to watch your son play catch with others because your arms and legs are paralyzed. Or not being able to speak due to brain damage. I want to shout right now but you can't hear me. PLEASE TAKE SAFETY AND PREVENTIVE HEALTHCARE SERIOUSLY!! *The best accident there is, is the one you prevent from happening. The best health condition is the one you caught early and beat or avoided altogether.*

We are back to our lovely—or not-so-lovely— game of Russian Roulette again. How many bullets does it take to blow your head off? ONE. How many four-wheeler rides without a helmet does it take to get seriously injured? How many stones in the eye to make you lose your sight? How many lightning bolts to critically injure you? How many boating trips without life preservers?... I think you see where I am going with this. STOP, PAUSE, and THINK.... What could happen if I don't take some preventive measures? What am I risking and most importantly—think really hard—is it worth it?

Ah, when you are young, you feel so invincible. (Now, if I sit down on a hard chair, I am afraid I am going to break my hip. That is not funny... well a little funny). Young people can charge life head on and not worry about anything. That is why in most high school yearbooks there are several pictures in the front in a section called, *In Memory Of.* My senior yearbook had several pictures in the front, many were baseball teammates of mine. They were not invincible, and neither are you or me.

I remember when I was in high school, I had a buddy who had an orange Camaro—Oh, I hope he is reading this book. We used to blast that seventies music and cruse all over the countryside. The faster and more reckless we went, the bigger the thrill it was. If we would have wrecked, all of life's thrills would have ended there. I'm sure you have heard the expression, 'NO FEAR'? Well, that will get us in trouble as well. If we do not fear the consequences, we will seldom think about safety.

Growing up in hilly Pennsylvania, sled riding was a very popular winter activity. My brother, friends, and I spent the day going up and down the big hills. Sometimes we would get to the top of a hill and could not tell how thick the trees were at the bottom. A few saplings are one thing to hit with a sled, but big trees were injuries waiting to happen. I remember, one time, we were exploring this new hill and it looked clear at the bottom. But just to make sure, we *SHOULD HAVE* walked down to check it out. The first kid down the hill soon found out that there are other things besides trees that can abruptly end a sled ride. This hill ended in a huge drop off into a creek. He yelled just in time for the rest of us to bail off our sleds. He got soaked, and was close to hypothermia by the time we got him to his house. But it could have been worse.

Now here is a thought for you. After you live a while, and have some personal experiences, (run over your foot with the lawn mower just once and you will be a different person cutting grass, trust me... I know), suddenly you become a lot more cautious. After I fell off the roof and broke my leg, I have slightly modified my roofing activities. When I think back to all the stupid things I used to do; well... I am shuddering now while writing about them.

Here I am painting my two-story house. (Guys, if you have ever done this, please don't tell wifey). Too cheap to get scaffolding or a good ladder, I took the old, wooden ladder I had and stood on the next to the top rung to get all but a little bit painted. To finish, (you may want to close your eyes. WAIT. Then you can't read any more...) anyhow, I duct taped a brush on the end of an old tomato stake and reached over and got that last section painted. Brave wasn't I? So courageous. *What an idiot!!!!* I would have never survived the fall onto the driveway unless I would have landed on my wife's van... then she would have killed me. (Can't win without safety).

So, whether you are a very, "It can't happen to me", type person or a young person who fears nothing, please remember that there are thousands of injuries and deaths which occur each year because of those two erroneous thoughts. Be serious about safety.

Sometimes, people are the same way with health issues. *"Nah, that's not important. I don't need that. That won't do me any good."* Well, let's ask Ted...

Ted was watching TV one night and heard a commercial for colon cancer screening. He was fifty-eight and the last time he saw his physician, which was five years ago, the doctor told him he should get a colonoscopy. Ted blew it off as he did the commercial. To him, he felt fine, and it *wasn't important.*

There was an interesting conversation that happened the next night at the supper table.

"Ted, do you remember Rita from the Miller's barbeque last week?"

"Ya, her husband's name is Earl."

"Yes, Barb Miller told me that poor Earl just found out he has late-stage colon cancer and there is nothing they can do. It has already spread to his liver and pancreas."

"Oh, my! That is horrible."

That was what Ted thought for a few minutes and then his mind quickly retreated to the doctor's advice and the television commercial. He now thinks that colon cancer screening is *important*. **QUESTION**: What if Earl had never gotten cancer or they would have never met Earl? Would Ted have put off the screening until it was too late? Would it be poor Ted in someone's conversation?

Take the time to be safe and take advantage of preventive healthcare screenings. You will get that time back in the long run. If you don't… the run might not be so long.

Chapter 4

Learn From Close Calls

One of the tragedies we learn from history is that we seldom change anything because of what we learn from history. The same applies to everyday life. We repeatedly make the same mistakes because we fail to allow those experiences to teach us that something needs to be changed. Be honest, have you ever done something, came close to a disaster but did the same thing again later on down the road?

Here is a good one that is not so bad. Have you ever hit your thumb with a hammer? It is a pain you just can't quite describe. It literally brings tears to your eyes. But wait, the pain begins to diminish, so you start back, and oh my goodness, you do it again and scream to the top of your lungs. Now man, that really hurts. But again, it will get better. Other cases are different.

Here is Neil. He is driving late at night and is very tired. He doesn't want to pull over because he wants to get home. Suddenly, he shakes himself and his eyes open when he hears a terrible noise—relax, he just hit the rumble strips. Now he is wide awake, alert, and feels like he can resume his trip. But that was a close call. What should it have taught him? Let's see... I'll pick you there in the recliner. What should it have taught him?... That is correct. (You think I'm a little nuts don't you. No worries, you're not alone). That's right sir; when you drive exhausted, you can fall asleep and not know it. So, what should that make him do? Right again. Pull over get some rest or at least walk around and get something to munch on or drink, but do not drive when you are drowsy.

But Neil here wanted to get home, so he continued on. Now we are back to leaving a whole lot to chance. The chance that he will never get home again, the chance he will never kiss his wife again, he will never hug those kids again—Neil, just pull over buddy, get home later, but get home.

You see, when we have close calls, we have two choices. Learn from them and change what you are doing or try it again and see if it is better the next time. I mean, I will be honest with you, I have had close calls and hate to admit it, I did the same thing again hoping for a different result. My rationale was: I learned something from what I was doing but I didn't learn that what I was doing could have had far worse results.

I have changed tons of electrical outlets. How many times have I gotten a little jolt? Ah, well, a few? Anyhow, I usually tell myself just to be more careful. Get this; even though I am being more careful, I am still not using available preventive measures to make sure it is safe. Flip the breaker to OFF.

One day, I was driving home from work in Pennsylvania. It was one of those days where it snowed in the morning, melted a bit in the afternoon, and started to freeze again just as I was getting off. (You know where this is going). I had to travel a pretty curvy road, so I started out slowly. The further I drove, seeing that the roads were OK, the faster I went. I got to the bottom of a hill, and there had been very wet, and now it was, ta da... ice. I did three doughnuts and finally stopped. I did not hit anything, and besides pointing the wrong direction, all was cool.

I really do hate telling this story because a few days later, I did the same thing; started out slow, sped up, and hit some ice. This time I smashed my little Geo Metro into a guardrail, and although, I was not hurt, Geo Metro vs guardrail is not even a contest: totaled. (I know, I should have just named this book, *"Just Don't Do What Allen Did and You'll Be Fine"*). I did not change my actions after that first close call, and it cost me.

Gina was driving down the road when she got a message. It was a friend who just wanted to say *'Hi'*, so she answered *'Hi'* back—yes, while she was driving. Well, the friend didn't know she was driving so she wrote her a novel. As Gina started reading the text which contained some pretty personal stuff, she got more into the text, and less into driving, until she heard a horn blaring. She had drifted into the other lane. She was able to correct herself and avoid the collision but what a close call that was. She started to sweat, and her heart was pounding wildly. She learned her lesson… or did she? She knew texting while driving was extremely dangerous, and that it has caused many fatal car accidents and almost another one. She learned, she realized, she saw, but did she *change*? *"I'll just text her back and tell her I can't text because I am driving."*—Gina, you have got to be kidding me. If you must do that, find a safe place to pull over and text till your fingers get all cramped up, but not while you are driving.

Close calls can also happen with your health. I have known several people who have had heart attacks but were able to recover after some treatment and rehabilitation and live normally. They may have resumed their normal lifestyles but that should have included some changes to prevent future heart issues.

"OK, you are doing fine now but I want to see you again in six weeks." (Didn't go… he felt fine) "I would like to see you lose about twenty pounds so follow the dietary instructions the dietitian gave you and follow the exercise plan the physical therapist started you on."

Well, he did follow that advice... for about a month. Then, back to his regular eating habits, got too busy again to exercise, and thus gained the weight back that he had lost. It takes a while to get over having a heart attack, so you are usually good for a little while. But wow, what a close call. Why don't we learn from them? Some people don't live through heart attacks.

George has to have skin cancers shaved off his head periodically, but has still doesn't wear a hat. Millie had a mini stroke, but hasn't quit smoking and doesn't get her blood pressure checked very often. Harry had several polyps removed that were borderline pre-cancerous, but he won't go back in for another colonoscopy. *Hey!!!!! What does it take?* Now if you don't care about your health or life, then don't worry about it but if you have things to do and people to live for, then please let the close calls teach you something.

I'll even go a step further. Are you ready and listening?... I mean, reading? We should also learn from the tragedies and close calls that others have had. When I was in elementary school, I lived on top of a huge hill. Down below was the town of Ford City, Pennsylvania. There were roads on either side of the town for traffic to get in and out of town but there was also a path and a set of steps through the woods which many people used to walk to downtown. Lots of kids rode their bikes down that same path too. One day, a young boy was going down the hill too fast, hit a tree, and was killed. Unfortunately, this is a true story.

I saw the tree he hit. I was only twelve, but it made quite an impression on me. I was always very slow and cautious riding down that path. For once, I did learn a lesson from someone else's tragedy.

Zack and Pete were friends. One time, they were white water rafting in separate rafts. Pete was in the lead, and for a while everything was fine, but then the wind began blowing and they came across some very rough water, lined with huge rocks. Zack was about fifty yards behind Pete but gaining speed. As he looked down the river, he saw Pete's raft get hit by a huge swell, thrown out of the water, turn over, and land on the rocks. Zach steered over towards the shore where the water was much calmer and looked for his friend. Pete was fine on the shore, with just a few bruises. Zach pulled his raft out of the water, right there and then. Hey Zach, you learned a great lesson the easy way. Prevention comes in many forms. Learning from the misfortunes of others can indeed be a great tool for prevention.

Karen called her friend Kelly to tell her that her neighbor's daughter had just gotten into the cleaning solutions under the kitchen counter. They rushed the child to the hospital, and he will be fine but boy, it was close. Both Karen and Kelly had latches installed on the cabinets where their cleaning supplies were stored. Good job, ladies... looks like we have some momentum going.

We don't like to see anyone get hurt or become ill, but if you can learn how to prevent what happened to them, take full advantage of it.

Chapter 5

Novice, Confident, Dangerous

This chapter will deal primarily with safety—wow, what a title for a chapter but as we start our discussion, you will see that the progression is spot on. Usually, when someone starts out on a new venture, they are extremely cautious. They are learning as they go so sometimes, they make a few mistakes, but they are not too serious. Then after a while, they have it down. They do everything right and are doing great. They are now very confident that they have mastered their new endeavor. That is where they reach a dangerous point because they feel that they are so good, they can modify the correct way to do it. And they don't need all that safety stuff anymore.

Joey got a new bike and is learning to ride it. He tips over a few times here and there, but he is just riding in his driveway, and he has his neat helmet on so it's no big deal. With each passing day, he gets better and better and starts riding to other places. He is still careful when he goes out onto the road, and he is still wearing his helmet. Then one day, Joey decided he is a pro at bike riding. He does wheelies, goes very fast, rides all over the place, and his helmet now stays in the house. He has just progressed from confident to dangerous. Then came the ramp jumping and riding with no hands on the handlebar. (Joey sounds a lot like all of us, doesn't he?)

Well, one day he was riding with no hands and no helmet. His balance was perfect, but he didn't see the rock that was in his way and—you guessed it, again (next book I write, I am going to call you all for some ideas since you know everything)—he fell, skinned up his knees and his arms, hit his head on the road, and the handlebar poked his stomach. No internal injuries, they watched him for a concussion and put dressings on his road rash. But it could have been much worse. We must be careful when we get confident so we don't neglect safety and become dangerous.

I bought a house a couple years ago and it has a couple acres of woods in the back and three fireplaces. So, guess what I got?—Aha! Stumped you that time, a chainsaw. It had been years since I used a chainsaw, so I started off doing things correctly, like starting it on the ground with my foot in the right place and wearing goggles and steel toes boots. But once I got the hang of it, it was tennis shoes, no goggles, and starting it improperly. I progressed to being dangerous. But since I started writing this book, I have reverted to confident and safe. (At least this book helped one person).

Here is the worst one, driving a car. When someone first gets their license, they are the safe and defensive drivers of the year. But as soon as they get a few hundred miles under their belt, all that safety stuff goes out the window. What did we learn about a traffic light turning yellow? The light was about to turn red, and traffic will be starting to come from another direction, right? Now it means you need to hit the gas so you can get through before the light turns red.

What does a yield sign mean? Nothing, the other guy will slow down and let you in. Do you still put your hands at the ten and two position on the steering wheel? No, just one hand anywhere on the wheel, and that is only when you aren't doing something; then you use your knee—I bet I got you on that one. No alcohol before driving; well not too much anyway. Always go the speed limit; at least, maybe a bit higher. Always buckle up... Ya, I have to do that to shut that noise off. Ever drive while distracted? I could hear a pin drop right now because you are all—not me now—you are all, well maybe occasionally, driving while doing other things.

I drive thousands of miles. I am on the road at least three days a week. I have seen people eating, (not just snacks, I mean quarter pounders), shaving, putting make-up on, talking on the phone, texting, husband and wife fighting, and a few times on my way to DC, I even saw people reading the newspaper. What on earth are they thinking? There is no way to give full attention to the road and the other vehicles while doing all those things. You watch the road just enough to stay between the lines, (kinda).

It's hard to be definitive with the stats because the causes of many accidents are unknown, but I guarantee you, many of them occur because the driver was preoccupied, causing untold numbers of injuries and fatalities.

I bought a car from a little Ma and Pop dealer a few years ago. He gave me a good deal and we really hit it off. He was just one of those nice guys. We talked about everything including how proud he was of his daughter. He told me to swing by anytime to just talk. He wasn't very busy, and we had a good time. About three months later, he was driving down a two-way road. A teenage girl, driving the other way, was changing CDs in her car, swerved over into his lane, and hit him head on. She lived, but he was killed instantly. I was in shock for a few minutes when I heard the news but then the tears came. I didn't know him well, but he was one of the good guys, and was killed by someone doing something terribly unsafe, (I had a different word to use there, but I thought it was best to keep the book PG), driving distracted. It was a senseless, preventable accident and fatality. Please take driving seriously. Vehicles traveling at 45–70 mph are lethal weapons; be sure to drive them carefully.

One of the worst things that can happen to someone who drinks and drives is getting to where they are going without getting caught. The first time they do it, it was after just a few drinks. They made it home safely so they developed more confidence that it wasn't a problem and they could still control their vehicle. The next time, they drank a little more and then a little bit more the next time. They never wrecked or got pulled over so now they never even think about it; they just do it. They are spinning the barrel on that pistol and each time they add a bullet. Sooner or later, it is going to go off.

People start boating very responsibly. I went fishing in a boat with a friend several times and he had a checklist. Oars in case the engine breaks down, *check*. Extra gas in case we run out, *check*. Fishing poles and bait, *check*. (Ah man, now I want to go fishing… hang on, I'll be right back). I wish you could see the size of this monster fish I caught. (No, I didn't measure it. Trust me it was big). OK, OK, where was I?... Life preservers; *check* and so on. Beer; *nope*, leave it for when we get back… smart call. Many start out that way, but soon, they are such confident boaters that they can go out without all the safety stuff. It may seem like a low figure, but it is estimated that over a hundred people are killed each year in boating accidents and many more are injured.

The irony is when people do things professionally, they are much more conscious of engaging safety measures. Mountain and rock climbers, scuba divers, pilots, and race car drivers all take safety very seriously and go to great lengths to make sure they are using all the necessary safety equipment.

Jerry always gets his car inspected at the same place every year. The garage he goes to has lost their inspection license several times for faulty inspection practices. But Jerry likes them because they just 'slap a sticker on'. He laughs and never worries about his car failing.

Here is a question for you Jerry... What if there is something terribly wrong with your car? Isn't that the idea of "safety inspections," to keep you "safe"? What if your brakes are bad and a little child runs out in front of you, and you must suddenly stop? What if you are going around some sharp bends on a mountainous road and the steering goes out? What if your tires are so bad that they fail to hold the road in heavy rain? It could be bye, bye Jerry and you may take some others with you.

Did you know that the NASCAR pit crews consist of five mechanics? They all are there to inspect and ensure the car is safe for the driver to operate. Think the professional car drivers will be taking their cars to your favorite garage, Jerry? Ya, I doubt it too. Think about it! Don't get so confident that you neglect safety.

Chapter 6

Don't Ignore the Warnings

People, institutions, departments, and groups have been very good about putting warnings in front of us. Unfortunately, these warnings get ignored which brings us to another huge subject in preventive health and safety; **don't ignore the warnings**.

I don't want to single anyone out, but I do want to give some illustrations of what I am referring to.

Look at these facts:

1. The Surgeon General has stated that cigarette smoking can be hazardous to your health.
2. Several medical agencies have confirmed that cigarette smoking is a major risk factor in many health conditions.
3. Insurance companies charge higher rates for smokers than non-smokers.
4. A very detailed warning is placed on every pack of cigarettes.
5. Still, although decreasing, roughly fourteen percent of the US population still smokes.
6. An estimated 440,000 people die each year from smoking related illnesses.

7. They estimate that the average smoker loses between fourteen to fifteen years of life expectancy.

OK, so now the question... are people ignoring the warning? Yes, indeed they are. Just think of how many lives could be saved and how many people would have fewer serious medical conditions if they would heed the warnings.

There is a continuous barrage of colon cancer screening commercials on TV, in pharmacies, hospitals, and most doctor's offices. Colon cancer, if caught early, can be treated. Late stages do not generally have a favorable prognosis. Why do so few people take advantage of these screenings? They ignore the warning.

Look at all the progress we have made with treating breast cancer. Again, breast cancer, along with most of the other medical conditions, can be treated successfully, if detected early.

We could go on and on about excessive alcohol intake, illicit and prescription drug abuse, unprotected sexual practices, continuous exposure to the sun, lead paint, carbon monoxide, leaving children and pets in hot vehicles, and so many more. Warnings, that if taken seriously, can be life savers but if ignored, can produce disastrous and lethal results.

Just a few comments now on overall health. The leading cause of death in the U.S. still is, and probably always will be, heart disease. This opens a huge opportunity to prevent you from developing it. What are some of the warnings out there which can help prevent heart disease? To reveal these, we just must look at some of the risk factors:

We have already mentioned smoking as a huge risk factor, so how about these other questions?

1. Do you get regular check-ups?
2. Do you get your cholesterol and triglyceride levels checked periodically?

3. Do you follow a diet that provides nutrition, but is mindful of excessive sweets, fats, and carbohydrates?
4. Are you maintaining a healthy weight and Body Mass Index? (I wanted to leave that one out for obvious reasons… I'm glad most of my pictures on the website are just head shots—no, I am not that big, but I can lose a few pounds).
5. Do you get all the procedures done that your doctor recommends like EKGs or a Stress Test?
6. Do you have a regular exercise program?
7. Have you been evaluated for sleep apnea?
8. Do you have ways to reduce stress?
9. Do you consume alcohol in moderation?

These things are very important to consider if you are trying to prevent heart disease. We hear about all of them, see advertisements, billboards, and ads everywhere to remind us about these things but heart disease still kills an average of about 800,000 people a year in the US alone—yes, you are right again, they ignore the warnings.

What about other warnings:

1. *Slow Down; Children Playing* – They are trying to get you to slow down because it is a neighborhood with lots of children out playing. Can you imagine failing to heed this warning and injure or kill a child? That would be hard to live with; especially after you saw the warning.
2. *Road Slippery When Wet* – How many accidents have there been because people didn't pay attention to this sign?

3. *Men Working or Work Area* – People working on the roads get hit all the time because someone tried to fly through a work zone.
4. *Hard Hat Area* – What can I say? It's your head.
5. *Buckle Up for Safety* – I sure hope I do not have to elaborate here. Seatbelts have saved thousands of lives when worn properly.
6. *Speed Limit Signs: Reduce Speed Ahead* – Speed limits are set by road design and location. They have reasons for wanting you to reduce your speed.
7. *Caution: Thin Ice* – Playing on the ice can be fun but it can also be deadly. Don't ignore this one.
8. *Railroad Crossings* – "Come on, hit it. If we hurry, we can beat the train!" You're not serious, right? Did you know that there are about 5,800 train/auto accidents each year? Most of these occurred at crossings and contributed to over 600 deaths. What are people thinking??
9. *Rip Tides* – Worldwide, drowning is the third leading cause of accidental deaths, averaging about 360,000 a year. The highest rates are from children aged one to four and then five to nine. Many of these were drownings due to rip tides.
10. *Weather Warnings* – "Well I took a chance and stayed, and nothing happened." Those four words should ring a loud bell. *I TOOK A CHANCE.* Why on earth would you leave your life up to chance? It is too risky. It was reported that in the U.S., there were over 580 deaths and over 1,700 injuries from weather-related incidents like hurricanes and tornados. That may not seem like many but it is if you or a loved one is one of them.

   A. *Hurricanes* – When they warn people to evacuate, please take their advice. When you are told to take shelter, you should do so. Many people don't and don't live to explain why. Don't forget, hurricanes may seem predictable, but several tornados can spin off a hurricane and they are very unpredictable.

B. *Storm warnings* – Many times during bad rain, ice, and snowstorms, people are warned not to travel because the roadways are hazardous. Remember we talked about the dangerous areas and chance? Don't go there because you ignore these warnings. What? You are going out to have fun on the road? You are endangering your life and the lives of the rescue team that has to get you out of your smashed vehicle.

C. *Heat Index and Freezing Temperatures* – These conditions are extremely dangerous for the elderly and those with health conditions. Many injuries and fatalities have occurred due to exposure of both heat and cold.

So, to wrap it up here, just make sure you don't ignore warnings whether they concern safety or health. Warnings are made for a reason. If there were no dangers involved, there wouldn't be warnings. The best warnings are the ones you take seriously, the most dangerous ones are the ones you ignore.

Stop, Pause, and Think

I want us to just stop, pause, and think about what we have discussed at so far. My book called, *Reincarnate Now*, basically deals with people who have regrets over things they did or didn't do in the past. Poor decisions and mistakes have cost them a lot and they would give anything to be able to go back and do it all over again, correctly.

I guarantee you that ignoring preventive health and safety will cause the same regrets, only for those who are fortunate enough to still be alive. The regrets kind of follow an "If–Then" format. *If* I had known I was going to get lung cancer, *then* I would have quit smoking years ago or never started. *If* I had known I was going to be paralyzed from the waist down, *then* I would have been more careful on the roof. *If* I had known that I was going to kill someone in a car accident, *then* I would have never tried to text someone while I was driving.

I could go on and on about tragedies that occur all the time which leave people with the most crippling regrets you can imagine. Bottom line: people get injured and sick, and yes, they die because they pay the high price of not engaging the ounce of prevention. Just one more staggering example: an average of 379 children drown in pools each year. About seventy-five percent of those are five years old or younger. Do you think there are some people who wish they would have had their pools more secured; or had watched their children more closely?

Please note this again; some of the figures I have presented seem rather low in comparison to the population. In this last case, the comparison doesn't really matter if it is your child or your pool. Stop, pause, and think about that.

Other things to remember:

1. When we do things subconsciously, we often neglect prevent safety measures.
2. Rushing and hurrying often causes us to skip employing safety measures. Engaging safety and preventive healthcare takes time, but it is well worth it.
3. The thought that, *"It won't happen to me"* or *"I won't get that"* are commonly very regrettable phrases.

4. We can't totally eliminate the risk, but we sure can reduce it.
5. People often get so busy; they fail to think about doing the things that will prevent injuries and the development of health conditions.
6. Remember the phrase, "You can pay me now (ounce) or pay me later, (a lot more)." Take that to heart.
7. Always compare what you are gaining, (making my tee-off time) to what you are risking, (losing an eye).
8. Taking advantage of preventive healthcare measures now will increase your odds for living longer and better lives.

Chapter 7

Safety for Infants and Small Children

We usually define infants as newborns up to one year old. Aren't they so beautiful and sweet? I worked in pediatrics for four years and thought every baby I saw was adorable. (I know, yours was the cutest. Actually, I think mine were—nah, I am not going to argue with someone that bought my book).

Although in the first couple of months, there doesn't seem to be too much of a need for safety, but there are some things to be aware of and this is a great place to start being, what I call, "safety conscious." In other words, it's a good time to start developing good safety habits. While the baby spends most of their time in the crib, seat, or bassinet, there isn't too much danger but the penny you dropped on the floor could cause problems once that little squirt starts crawling all over the place. Start the habit of making sure the floors are free of any objects they could place in their mouths.

But for our newborns, we can think of a few things to remember. Well, let me ask you this question; how long should you heat up a baby bottle in the microwave? Answer: DON'T EVER WARM UP A BABY BOTTLE IN A MICROWAVE. It has been proven that formula heated in the microwave can have "hot spots" and they could be dangerous for that little baby. So, the FDA recommends that you don't do it. You can buy several thermometers and other temperature-checking monitoring devices but to be FDA safe, take those extra few minutes and bypass the microwave.

Some parents laugh as they talk about putting the baby into their little seat, reclining it, and propping the bottle into their mouths. Let's go back a bit. Remember I said that safety measures decrease the risk involved in an action? Well, propping the bottle is not a safety measure and not a good practice. Why would a parent do that when they can hold that sweet little thing? I'll tell you why, they want to multitask. *"I can feed the baby and do (insert task here). I am right there with them."* You can multitask a lot of things but don't do it with your baby. Cherish that feeding time. It is good for you and for them.

When they get a bit older, you obviously have to be more careful as they develop the ability to roll over and scoot around a bit. They should never be laid on a bed, couch, changing table, or other elevated surface without hands-on attention. The Center for Disease Control (CDC) states that fifty percent of non-lethal injuries in infants under one-year- olds are due to falls. Please, please, please, stop, pause, and think before you leave your baby in potential danger.

We talked earlier about the penny on the floor; well somewhere around six to eight months, those little darlings start putting everything in their mouths. It starts with hands and feet and then progresses to anything and everything they can find. And once they are able to start picking things up, you need to have eyes installed into the back and sides of your head. Those little rascals are quick, aren't they? (Until they start getting old enough to do chores, and then mysteriously, they get really slow).

As the infants start crawling, they open themselves up to a whole new world of things to explore and additional danger areas as well. In the average house, guess what is just about at eye level of crawling children? Yes indeed, electrical outlets. These are more dangerous as children get a little older, but as soon as they are mobile on the floor, it's time to take action. I know what you are saying, *"I would never let my child crawl around on the floor if I was not right there with them."* Yes, that is our intention but you and I both know things come up. It was noted in 2016, that over 2,400 children were injured by electrical outlets. That is more than enough to make me think seriously about prevention. Remember, the more attention you pay to prevention—hey that rhymes—the lower the risk factors are.

At this point, most parents rush out and get the plastic outlet covers. Temple University did a test study and a hundred percent100% of the two- to four-year-old children were able to get the plastic covers off of the outlets. That means they are not the best preventive measures, and the risk has not been reduced. That is why the National Electric Code recommends the use of Tamper Resistant Receptacles (TRRs). I know, you hate those things because sometimes it is hard to put plugs into them. Well, you will love them the first time you look over at your pride and joy messing with an outlet. An ounce of prevention...

Oh, let me add one more thing here... PLEASE pay extra close attention when visiting grandma and grandpa or other people's houses because chances are, their houses may not be childproof, especially if they do not have any young children.

Not only do you have to consider what they are doing, you also have to think about where they are going. That means doors should be closed and gates placed in front of passageways that do not have doors. Do not leave any stairs unguarded, this means up or down because they can be a real hazard to crawling or walking children.

Here is another one. While working for EMS, I cannot tell you how many times I responded to a child who had their head stuck in the rungs of a staircase. I do not know how it happens. You would think that if they can slide their head through it, they could also slide it back out but somehow their heads grow when they are stuck—ya, I know it sounds funny—and they won't come back out. We did get them out without too much effort. Did you know Crisco is a required item in ambulances now? (Did you really believe that?) No, we just borrowed it or baby oil to lube the tyke up a bit and then, POP, all is well.

I suppose now is as good as time as any to bring the next point up; watch your children around pets. Now, most of the time, pets and little children get along pretty well, but small children like to hit and pull hair and tails, and sometimes, that particular pet may be having a bad day and you do not want to take a chance on a bite or scratch injury. Some dogs will get aggressive if someone bothers their feeding time or while they are chewing on something. Cats can scratch and after walking around in the litter box, you can imagine their claws are not very sanitary—look up cat scratch fever.

I will not go over other pets but just be careful when your little ones are around them. Just a thought about dogs though; in 2016 it was reported that about fifty percent of all children under twelve years old had been bitten by a dog. Dog bite injuries totaled more than *bike accidents, playground injuries, moped, skateboard, and ATV injuries.* Not all of these were inflicted by their own pets, but many were.

Another thing to consider is that babies who crawl all over the place get very dirty hands. I can see some of the ladies getting a bit red in the face. *"Are you saying my house is dirty?"* No, but come on, you know what I am saying. No matter how clean your house is, floors were not designed for cleanliness, especially if you have pets. The recommendations: wash those little hands often, especially before they eat, and have handwipes all over the house so clean up is quick and easy.

I have to tell this story because I love telling it. When my first son was around four years old, I took him with me to view a building I was looking at for a meeting place. It was vacant and hadn't been used for seven to eight months. I was talking to the perspective landlord and noticed my son was chewing something.

I said, "What are you chewing buddy?" He answered, "Gum."

"And where did you get that gum?" (You already know what he said don't you?).

"Under that table, there."

Man, I washed his mouth out and brushed his teeth and made him gargle for an hour. Trust me, wash their hands often.

About the same time they start motoring all over, they also start pulling themselves up on things and standing up in the crib and playpen. You will find with each developmental step comes more chances for injuries. Yeah, they can stand, but they can fall too. It is also a good time to identify all the things they may be able to pull off a table or shelf. Dangling chords are very inviting to those little tikes.

Let's consider this scenario before we start on falls. You thought that it would be nice to put the baby's crib close to the window for the light and so they could see outside. One day you walk in, and your baby is all wrapped up in a small cord... the pull cord for the blinds. Thank goodness everything was OK, but can you imagine how it could have turned out? Be a good Chief Inspector and find every potential danger around your baby and prevent any accidents from occurring.

Babies just don't show up one day and say, "Hey, I am moving in." (And sometimes they don't seem to ever say, "Hey, I am moving out." either). Anyhow, that means you have time to prepare. Look over the house and plan for the baby's arrival.

As they hit that walking stage, it is very important to identify all the things they can pick up, (picked up that penny yet?), reach, and all the things they could hit if, when, they fall.

I know coffee tables and end tables with glass tops look nice and the glass is strong, but they can also pose a safety issue. Tables usually have corners and those can also be dangerous. You can't change all your furniture nor take everything out of the room that has corners, I am just saying be mindful of things which could cause an injury.

Every parent has heard that horrible sounding *'thud'* and the ensuing screaming of a small child who has fallen and hit their head on something. It comes with that age group, and they seem to bounce right back but we should do everything we can to avoid injuries. (Ha, ha, can you picture those little ones walking around with a helmet on?). How many times have you heard, *"You've got to watch those toddlers like a hawk"*? Even that is an understatement.

Man, by time we get done with this section on children, we can see why parents are nervous wrecks by time the kids go to school. As their eating habits change, you know that choking can become an issue. I hear parents boasting all the time of how quickly their children progress up to regular foods. You cannot teach a two- to three-year-old to chew their food sixteen times or not to put too much food in their mouths. They inevitably also like to walk, talk, and laydown while they are eating. These can all cause the child to accidently get food lodged in their windpipes causing them to choke.

Sometimes it can be cleared easily with a couple coughs but sometimes it is not so easy. Over 10,000 children below the age of fifteen are treated in emergency departments each year due to chocking. Of those, an average of seventy-five fatalities take place. The main culprits are hot dogs, believe it or not. We give them to our little ones because they are soft and easy to chew— and they love them, well who doesn't?). The big problem is that pieces of hot dog fit very well into a child's airway. If you give small children hot dogs, cut them up well and avoid just slicing them once crossways.

Going back to even smaller children for a second, we also have to think about the things we give them to play with once they are old enough to hold things. Remember where almost everything goes? Correct, into the mouth. Years ago, the dolls used to have eyes which came off and toys had so many pieces which could be pried off and would then end up in children's mouths.

Even though there have been many added regulations and changes made in the toy industry, parents must remain the last line of defense to ensure toys and other handheld things are safe for their children. I am sure you have noticed that most toys now come with clearly marked ages listed for who the toy is most appropriate for. There are other reasons for those age listings besides cognitive ability and one vulnerability is choking.

I love to surf fish. You get everything set up and if the tide is coming in—best time to fish—you have to keep moving your stuff a little further back, that is always so fun. It seems like we do that with children as well. As they get taller and can reach higher, we have to keep looking at all the things they can possibly get their mitts into.

One day you will notice that there is nothing around under your waist level and all the higher shelves and mantles are packed with everything. Oh, the fun of parenting. I am doing similar things now because of a German Shepard "puppy" that is huge and tears up everything. Sometimes I say that I would rather have another baby. But then…

Obviously, the kitchen is a very crucial place to watch. Get in the habit early of not leaving knives laying around on lower counters and ensuring that none of the pot or pan handles are where they can be reached and pulled down. Oh, and look here… there are doors under the sink and inside are a bunch of cool looking bottles full of pretty-colored liquids—yes, you know where I am going. Any reachable cabinet should have a child-proof locking mechanism so children cannot reach the contents. (I know, some of you ladies are wondering if hubby will be able to get in there now). As a double safety measure, it is also suggested that poisons like cleaners and furniture polishes should be stored behind locked doors in area which is totally off limits to children, like a utility room or closet with a locking door.

I could go on and on but the most important point I am trying to make is that safety doesn't happen by accident, and it seldom comes while we are just winging our way through life. It takes deliberate thinking, conscious awareness, keen observation, and planning. As I mentioned before, even with all preventive measures in place accidents still happen and tragedies still occur. That is just a part of life.

I heard from a neighbor once about a family down the street. The six- and eight-year-old boys were playing ball in the yard. Their father got a distressing call from work, and while still on the phone, he jumped into the car to go and check things out. In a hurry to get there, he put the car in reverse and quickly started backing down the driveway. He stopped in just a few seconds in total horror as he felt the car running over something and heard screaming.

He slammed the car into park and jumped out, dropped his phone as he could see his six-year-old son under the car, bleeding and barely moving. He immediately called 911 as people rushed from all over to try and help. They were able to get the boy out but by then it was too late.

I lost a twenty-year-old son back in 1999. I still miss him terribly today and when it happened, I didn't think I could live through it. I can't imagine losing a child knowing that I caused it to happen, or I didn't do something which could have prevented it. Please think seriously about safety. I don't want you to have to live with suffocating regrets.

Chapter 8

Raising Safety Conscious Children

As we progress to the older children, we are going to add something. When little children reach for the stove, we attempt the best way we can to get them to understand that they are not to do that. We usually try to explain in technological terms like, *"No, no, no, hot, burny, burny, no, no, no."* I teach leadership and motivation and one of my big points is to "Teach the *WHY.*" Well, with this age group, you kind of have to settle for trying the best you can to convince them that it's burny, burny.

However, when they get older and have a slightly better understanding of the situation, it's time to teach them the *WHY* and start teaching them about safety consciousness or translated, "being careful." I am telling you this for a fact; if we can get children, and older people too, to equate safety and preventive healthcare to keeping terrible things from happening, they will be much more meaningful.

"Mom, I don't want to wear that stupid helmet when I am riding my bike. None of the other kids do."

Sound familiar? Now you can say:

"Because I am your mother and I said so. I don't care what other mothers allow their kids to do."

Wow, now that really does sound familiar. Have you Moms said that?... Come on, fess up.

So, now you need to do some research and planning. Statistics tell us that about 1,000 children a day are treated in emergency rooms for bicycle accidents. Many of those are head and neck injuries and eighty-eight percent of those with head and neck injuries occurred because they were not wearing helmets, and yes, these accidents often cause fatalities and permanent brain damage. Now, your job is to digest that and explain at their level *how the brain can get injured, what that injury can cause,* and *why it is important to wear that helmet.* You know, with the internet available, we have no excuses for not doing a thorough job training for our children to be safety conscious and take advantage of preventive healthcare.

Johnny likes to play with matches. Look up the stats on how many children get injured from playing with fire, show them pictures of children who have been burned, a house burning down, and a forest fire. You see, you are teaching them that playing with fire is wrong, but you are also showing them why.

Jerry and his friends play right next to the road all the time and often, just run right out onto it. Same as above, do some research, show them some pictures, and warn them about what horrible things could happen if they keep playing close to the road and running out onto it.

We have talked about rushing and being too busy for safety. Don't rush this. Take the necessary time to properly warn them of the possible danger. Besides that, what do you think will make more of an impact; the process we just described or yelling out the window, *"Get away from that road!"*? They will sense that it is important if you take the time and really focus on their understanding.

We could go over so many more scenarios. In fact, I could probably do a couple chapters just on some of the crazy stuff I did as a kid. But here is the ask. Start teaching them to *stop, pause,* and *think* before they do something which could be dangerous. I am not going into the deep teachings on self-preservation, but I do believe we have a mechanism inside of us that warns us when we are doing something which can be dangerous.

Some people call it a "thrill." *"I was going eighty miles per hour on that back country road. What a thrill."* It is an adrenalin rush that comes when we are frightened or aware of danger. When I worked on roofs in the past, I always got that, feeling or sensation which made me just a little more cautious. Sometimes we rush and override that feeling and that is when we can get into trouble. Start climbing to the top of a tree and see as the limbs get smaller, note how you feel about going higher. We just need to teach them when those feelings come, think about how safe it is with what they are doing, and what you can do to make it safer. Then also, know their routines, what they do, and look for areas of potential danger.

Kim and Annie are en years old, live in town, and walk three blocks to school every day. So there you have, *watch the road, be careful in the crosswalks, wait for the traffic police to wave you through,* and *never talk to strangers, especially anyone pulling up beside you in a car*—and don't forget all the *WHYs*).

Most of us parents are worrywarts when it comes to some things but please take safety seriously and do all you can to train your children to be safety conscious. You will never know what you could be preventing but you will be so glad you did.

Sometimes, we parents turn out to be softies.

"Mommy, can you buy me that candy bar?" "No, honey, you have enough candy at home." "But I like that kind, please."

"No, Sherri, let's go."

"Please Mommy, I'll be real good." "Oh, ok, bring it here."

"Thanks Mommy! Mommy, can we stop for ice cream on the way home?" (Ha ha ha ha. You softie you!).

Now if this was a book written by parenting experts, they would probably say that we should not have given in. Personally, I would have only given in if it was a candy bar that I liked so I could get a bite, and I wanted ice cream too—I know, bad Daddy! But the point is, candy and ice cream are one thing but with safety, do not budge an inch.

"Daddy, can I sit on your lap and pretend I am steering while you drive?"

"Sure, little fella, hop up here and let's go."

Isn't that just so cute? It is also one of the most dangerous things you could possibly do with a child in a car. So very nicely say no, explain why it is so dangerous and what could happen if there was an accident.

"Mommy, can I go swimming over at Kathy's?" "Are her parent's home?"

"No, but her older sister is home and she can watch us." "Let's wait until Kathy's mom gets home."

"Ah, come on, please, pretty please, we will be good, and we never go near the deep end. Please!"

(They can be so persuading, can't they?)

"Mom, can I ride bikes with Ryan down to the little store?"

"Your dad said he wanted to go riding with you first so he could show you some things about safe riding on the road."

"But Mom, Ryan is here, and he rides down there all the time."

"Your dad will be home in about half an hour. You can wait."

"Ah come on, please mom. I will be really careful."

Many times, the kids will win the battles but stand your ground when it comes to safety. You don't want to be saying later on down the road: *"I told him he should wait; I shouldn't have given in. This is all my fault."*

Chapter 9

Danger! Danger! We Have a Teenager

Every stage of human development brings with it a different set of safety risks. It ranges from making sure the baby doesn't fall off the changing table to the elderly not falling and breaking a hip. When the teenage years hit, the risks seem to peak.

The CDC states that forty-eight percent of all teenage deaths are due to unintentional injuries. Non-fatal injuries also leave many teenagers paralyzed or permanently disabled. This is a good place to emphasize how important it is for parents to really focus on safety *WITH* their teenager. The ideal thing to do would be to take a leave of absence from work and stay by their side twenty-four-seven, but as we know, that isn't possible. Or we can keep them in locked rooms until they are over twenty but again, unrealistic. We could go the Big Brother route with GPS tracking devices but there again, it wouldn't really work. Not allowing them to drive while they are teenagers may also help but you'll have a huge fight on your hands until they get their license. The most effective ways to help prevent teenage accidents are INSTILLING in them just how important safety is.

One way would be to have them read this book. (Get one for all your children, nieces, nephews, friends, grandkids, and neighbors—free advertising at its best. Ha ha!). Seriously though, I am hoping that by the time you are finished with this book, you will be able to teach and train your children, at every age, just how important safety really is.

Many teenage accidental deaths each year are caused by falls, drownings, electrocution, and fires. An ever-growing number of teenagers die each year from accidental overdoses of illicit and prescription drug use. Drug use certainly has become an epidemic of massive proportions among our young. I will not get preachy here, and this isn't a book on raising children, but MOST drug abuse begins with associations. Not many teenagers just decide one day to start using drugs; they are usually introduced to drugs by an acquaintance. You don't necessarily need to hire a private detective, but it is good to know as much as possible about those who they associate themselves with.

Just a few other thoughts on the vital task of teenage safety promotion:

1. Again, don't rush this. Yelling *"Be careful!"* as they run out the door isn't what I consider safety training. It may be better to do several thorough segments than a few hour-long dissertations.

2. Talk objectively and ask them open ended questions. Don't just ask questions that they can answer with *yes* or *no*. Please do not turn into a college professor or psychiatrist here. *"Tell me about the things that you encounter each day that could present you with safety risks."* (Mom, are you OK? Ha ha). They are the love of your life and have been with you for nine months plus however old they are Mom—Dads, subtract the nine months. Just talk to them. *"Honey, you know how*

important safety is to us. We don't want any bad accidents to happen in our family. What things do you think you might have to be really careful about doing?"—Something like that.

3. You can talk to them about specifics too, like walking to school, watching out for traffic, not talking to strangers, staying away from drugs, and other things which may be specific to them.

4. Always review with them the relationship between safety measures versus risk and outcomes. *"Can you imagine losing an eye, or being confined to a wheelchair, or having brain damage and just lying in a bed all your life?"*

5. Share internet facts and pictures with them. *"This boy here was playing in an old, abandoned building. A board broke and he fell three stories and broke his neck and back. He died instantly but no one found him for two days."* Stories like that may open some eyes.

6. Bring things up casually as well as at sit down sessions. While you are listening to the news, *"Oh my, did you hear that? Two teenage girls were skating on the river, and they went out to where the ice was thin, fell through, and they still haven't found them."*

7. Make sure the conversation relays care and love, knowing the risks they face every day.

8. Make sure you are consistent, providing short, constant reminders so they know you are serious.

Teaching teenagers about safety will take time and patience. There are several things that you, as a parent, also need to think about. Many people have guns in the house, and they can be dangerous for little children who may accidently stumble across them. Teenagers, for various reasons, will actually look for them. They may have no malice intentions to use them, but many teenagers are injured and killed each year handling firearms that were in the house. Keep them locked up and have trigger locks on them so they cannot be fired.

I know you are wondering how good a gun is for protection when it is locked up or has a trigger lock on it. There are locks and lock boxes that allow both easy access with a short code but ensures only those who have the code can open it. Do some research. There are more accidental shootings in the home than there are with gun owners using a gun to ward off criminals from breaking in.

And how about the liquor cabinet? I am not saying at all that no one should have one or that a drink here or there is bad; but I am saying, when it's in the wrong hands, liquor can be deadly or cause injuries. I don't think, like a weapon, you would need emergency access, (unless it was a really bad day), so keep that alcohol under lock and key.

We were discussing drug overdoses earlier. I hate to say it but not all drugs taken are from the streets. Some were found right there in the medicine cabinet. It is understandable for people with chronic pain to have narcotics in their homes, but in the wrong amount, again in the wrong hands, can be fatal. CDC Vital Signs states that over 15,000 people die each year from overdosing on *PRESCRIPTION* drugs. That is more than cocaine and heroin overdoses combined. Please make sure your prescription medications are also locked up securely.

Now I am sure many of you, as you were reading over the liquor, guns, and prescription drug sections were saying, *"My child would never do that."* I have two words for you…

PEER PRESSURE. Many children do things they would not normally do because of peer pressure or because they are trying to impress others. It seems to be a bigger problem for those with lower self-esteem. They try to elevate their status by doing something grandiose like walking around with one of dad's guns or offering some alcohol to their friends. Your children may not ever do anything like that, but still do your part to ensure things that need to be locked up are locked up.

We touched on this earlier, but I can't stress enough how important it is for your teenagers to realize how fragile life is and that they are not indestructible. I can remember several times—and I bet you can as well—doing some really foolish things that were very dangerous. They could have easily ended my life or changed it in a very horrible way. I thank God that I am still here today and able to plead with others to value safety more than thrills and excitement.

Just one story and then a few comments on it. (It is really horrible that I have so many to choose from. I was a mischievous and reckless teenager). When I was sixteen, I got a bow and enjoyed shooting it at a target I had on a few bails of straw. My friend would come over and we would shoot together for a while. One day, I shot an arrow straight up in the air just to see where it would land. It seemed to be really cool until the sun started getting in our eyes and we couldn't follow the arrows. So, there we were, *"One, two, three, SHOOT."* Two arrows going up and neither of us could see where they were coming down. We did stare up in the sky watching for them—wow, it gives me tremors now just thinking about it. Where could one of the arrows have hit? (Yep, you are right). I can use this word now because I am referring to me… what a stupid thing to do. *What on earth was I thinking?* Aha, well that is the point… I wasn't thinking at all, just doing.

Now we go back to Chapter 1… We were *NOT* thinking; just winging it. Just doing our thing without thinking about the risk or possible consequences. That is why so many teenagers die from unintentional accidents and more are seriously injured. *Stop, pause, and think!* Training your children to do this can save them from so much danger and save you from so much grief. It's not easy but start early, be consistent, and soon it will be a part of their character. That is not saying they will never do anything dangerous, but it will decrease their chances of doing it.

Obviously, it would be easy to devote an entire chapter to auto safety. But let's just say for now that auto accidents take more teenage lives than any other type of accidents. It will be easier to stress safe driving if they have already gotten several years of how important safety in general is.

Now, I hope there will be several young people reading this and if that is you, please take to heart the things we have discussed. Life is wonderful and you have your whole life ahead of you. Just make sure it isn't cut short because of something that you could have prevented. Cool is cool but alive is better. If you are now driving, you know you are supposed to keep the car between the lines. Draw some safety lines and stay between them. Don't swerve out of the safety lane or let anyone talk you into doing it either because once you leave safety, you enter into a danger zone where risk and bad things await.

Chapter 10

Adult Safety

This will be a really short chapter because all of us adults know everything about safety and are safety conscious every day... *Because of the false nature of the last statement, I am compelled to write a slightly more in this chapter.* Accidents are the third leading cause of deaths in adults accounting for over 173,000 deaths per year. A couple of the major contributors are of course, automobile accidents and believe it or not, drug overdoses. Again, we will discuss automobile safety in a separate chapter.

To review from the first chapter, we discussed doing so many things subconsciously and when we do that, we often do not think about safety. At various life stages, this problem escalates and many adults encounter accidents, even fatal ones, because of it. The fifth leading cause of unintentional accidental deaths is choking. How can choking be a major player in accidental deaths? I am not going to go over the basic mechanisms of chewing, swallowing, and breathing but let's just say that if not done correctly, you will choke. If the piece of food is large enough and gets lodged in hard enough, you could die.

Here is Glen. He is a really hard worker and a great supervisor. He buys some food for his team and asked if they could have a working lunch. What do you do during a working lunch? You eat and work. How are these folks working? They are discussing next year's budget. The meeting starts to get a little intense while everyone is chewing, swallowing, and talking. Kyle decides to interrupt someone as he wants to make a point. So, he takes a deep breath… with a partially chewed meatball in his mouth and… yep, you guessed it…

My mom used to tell us all the time, *"Don't talk with food in your mouth."* She was pretty smart. And you think, *"I do it all the time."* Well, most of the deaths are from children choking but the adults who have died from choking probably made that same statement at some point. Any guesses as to why they teach how to aid a choking victim with CPR now? Because it happens so often. Just be conscious of it. By the way, Kyle never did get to make his point.

Here is another case. Henry has a bunch of friends over to watch the Pittsburgh Steelersand the Bengals. They are eating and having a great time when the Steelers return a kickoff, to the 50, the 40, the 30, the 20, the 10 and Henry jumps up and yells, "TOUCHDO—" That is all he got out. Yes, right again… he choked. But they did the Heimlich Maneuver on him, and he was fine, learned a great lesson, and by the way, the Steelers beat the Bengals, again, as always.

Older adults also have more issues with choking. Some of that could be due to problems with their teeth or just their ability to swallow. Like children, smaller bites are advisable as is adequately chewing their food before attempting to swallow. It is also important to make sure their mouth and throat do not get too dry. Again, it's probably not best to carry on too much of a conversation if they have choking issues.

Falls are another major cause of injuries and fatalities. Before we reach our elderly years, most of those falls are preventable and are due to a lack of safety prevention at work and at home. I mean, how can you just fall off a roof—OOPS!

I already told you that story. And it is a story filled with total disregard for safety. It often goes back to just not thinking about the dangers involved in what we are doing and ignoring various warnings. We have discussed several of those already, but think about it; what does it really mean to be "safety conscious"? Easy, just stop, pause, and think before you do things. And don't classify things as "non-dangerous" just because you see no immediate dangers.

On a very cold January day, I had a board meeting in a hospital. After the meeting, one of the board members shook my hand and excused himself because he had another meeting that he had to hurry to. I left a few minutes later, and as I exited the hospital, I saw four people looking down at the ground near the parking lot. Sure enough, there was the board member. He had hurriedly walked across some ice, fell, and hurt his back. It wasn't serious, but it certainly could have been a lot worse. Walking isn't particularly dangerous, but wait, there are some icy patches out here, I better be careful.

Other times it's just a matter of being willing to take risks. *"Let's take the boat closer to the dam. That's where the big fish are," "You don't need a helmet to ride a four-wheeler. The ground is soft," "I know it's not legal to hunt at night, but that is when the deer come out," "I've been in this bucket truck tons of times. I don't need that harness."* I guarantee thinking like that can, and does, cause accidents and fatalities.

As we grow older, our bones become more brittle and susceptible to fractures. A seemingly simple fall on the back side can mean a hip fracture for elderly people. Catching themselves with their hands can cause a variety of upper extremity fractures. The CDC states that about every second, an elderly adult is injured or killed from a fall. It is the number one cause of injury in the elderly. There are many precipitating factors that can produce falls, and the prevention is based on the reason for the risk. Loose steps and uneven sidewalks may be easily navigated for the young—fix both anyways—but they can pose problems for the elderly. Some elderly people are not as steady on their feet due to inner ear problems, medications, and even visual impairments. It is not a shame to need a walker or at least a cane to help steady you. It is much better than falling and getting badly injured. Sometimes, those of us who are getting up there in years have a pride thing going on and we don't want to admit we need a little assistance with something as simple as walking. But again, an ounce of prevention is worth not falling.

Here is another good place to park for a bit. I can remember at many different ages falling in the bathtub or shower. It can get very slippery, and if it isn't a walk-in shower, just stepping over the side of the tub to get in can cause more risk for a fall. *"Well, I don't like mats in the bathtub. They get yucky. And I don't like the little things you stick on the bottom of the tub either."* Well, do you like body casts, hospital stays, and traction? I didn't think so. Mats and the non-slip stickers can be cleaned fairly easily. Bones take a bit more time and effort to heal. Handrails are also great in showers and bathtubs. Just having something to hold onto helps support you as you get in and out. As a matter of fact, they are also quite helpful at the top of stairs, in entry ways, and in other places you may have to shift a lot of your weight to climb up or down.

Again, I have to keep reiterating—there is my one big word for you. I try to have at least one per book—but I, in no way, cover all the details. I am sure you can and will come up with so many more. Now just an example. As I was typing that, I was thinking; you should never put sharp knives in soapy dishwater. You can't see what is in there because of the suds so you could very easily get cut. Put them is a safe place on the sink and wash them separately. See how easy it is to think: *Prevention.* (Now guys, if you don't help with the dishes, there may be another type of injury heading your way. Think prevention… unless the football game is already on, then just risk it).

Chapter 11

Safety at Home

I have already stated that we cannot possibly cover every safety topic in this book. There are many other good books out there and I am sure it would be worth your time to read them too. However, I do want to cover some things in the home that we also need to look at.

We have discussed switching breakers off before working on electricity and using the special child-proof outlets but in general, always respect electricity. If you have an older home, it wouldn't hurt to have the wiring, outlets, and switches checked by a professional. I know, *"Do you know how much that costs?"* But I will answer your question with another question: "Do you know how many house fires are caused by electrical fires?" Thirty- six percent of house fires in the US are due to electrical issues; that is over one third. Believe me, a professional inspection will be well worth the cost. You must know by now... *An ounce of prevention.*

Additionally, be observant and do not think anything is too trivial to worry about. *"The outlet sparks slightly when I pull the plug out," "The switch sparks when I flip the light on, the wiring is pulling out of that lamp," "I can see a little bare wire on that extension cord," "The wall is very warm around that outlet."* On and on we could go, just remember to respect electricity. It is great for all the things we use it for but it can be very harmful if we treat it badly.

Fires

While we are on the subject of fires, in 2018, 2,620 deaths were reported from house fires in the U.S. I know it seems like a small number, but if it was someone you knew or loved, it is a huge number.

Obviously not all fires can be prevented. The three main causes of house fires are cooking/kitchen fires, heating units, and electrical problems. (Did you hear that? I heard someone say, "*Me and the kids love it when Mama burns supper. Saves us from a lot of suffering and we get to eat out."*). Shame on you sir. Anyhow, burning supper is one thing; however, burning the house down from a kitchen fire is quite another.

Kitchen fires can be nasty and they can spread very quickly. We will discuss extinguishing fires a little later but one reason kitchen fires become so bad is because people think throwing water on any fire will put it out. But in kitchens, grease is involved, which it makes it worse.

Now, I know you won't admit is but let me ask you a few 'Kitchen Fire' questions:

1. Have you ever turned on your stove and left it unattended for a while and FORGOT you had it on?— *Come on now, fess up.*
2. Have you ever caught a potholder or a tea towel on fire because it touched the burner as you were getting a pan off?—*I've been there too.*
3. Do you occasionally read directions on how high to turn burners up? *"I'm hungry, crank that fire up, and get that bacon frying."* (High temperature and grease and hurry = disaster).

4. Ever get a little too close and catch some of your clothes on fire?

If you answered *Yes* to any of these, you are probably more honest than the rest. (Ha ha). Sometimes, it's those, "Oh shoot, burnt the potholder" and sometimes, it's a 911 event. So, please be careful in the kitchen.

Heating units also use a lot of electricity which can often cause fires. I personally have seen a melted heater cord, and had it been in a different location, it could have caused a fire. Fireplaces, wood stoves, and other open heating methods must be watched carefully. It is imperative that you spend time reading up on how to operate them properly and safely. And once you get the hang of it and everything goes well, don't attempt to take shortcuts, or try new things which are not safe. It only takes one fire to burn a home and injure or kill those inside.

Those of you who smoke or allow smoking in your home, please do it safely and never, ever smoke while you are drowsy or could easily fall asleep. Never smoke in the bed either. Too many fires have started and too many lives have been lost from that very scenario.

Dryer fires are also a cause of many fires, so make sure you:

1. Clean the lint filter every load or two. Do at least one check every load.
2. Take the lint filter out and, using your narrow shop vac attachment, clean out the chamber below the filter.
3. Check and clean out all the lint from behind the dryer, making sure the exhaust hose is well connected.
4. Clean the exhaust hose out occasionally. (Depending on the amount of use).
5. Check to ensure your dryer is venting properly to the outside.

6. Remove the outside cover and clean inside as far as your attachment will reach.
7. Make sure the electrical cord is securely plugged in and that there is nothing near the outlet.

We can't skip past Christmas. Real Christmas trees are cool but if they dry out and you have the wrong type of lights, it creates the potential for a horrible Christmas for you and your family. It seems like the holidays are also a big time to see how many extension cords can be run and connected to only one or two outlets. It would be beneficial to do some research on the proper use of extension cords. Most tags on appliances and extension cords will tell you about possible fire dangers. (What, you never read those tags? I am shocked. I was sure you, for one, would read them).

Ok ladies, you can relax a little now. Guys, you have to keep the basement and garage cleaned up. Chemicals and oily rags are fires waiting to happen. And Barbeque Bill, please don't leave the grill unattended for long, especially if it is on a patio or even close to the house.

Rounding it up, watch what you burn inside a home. Candles and incenses are nice but they do get lit, and they can cause fires.

Okay, so let's ask some questions in case you do happen to have a fire:

1. Do you check to make sure your smoke detectors are working and change the batteries every six months? (Most people change batteries on July 4th and Christmas or New Years, just to remember). Whenever you do it, don't forget. Write it on your new calendar when you put it up.
2. Look at the condition of your fire extinguishers and read the gages every month. (I know, you are saying

that is an overkill, but you want it to work properly if you need it, right? Come on, it only takes ten seconds.) They should be tested every year but truthfully, as inexpensive as the small ones are now, buying new ones is another option. The larger ones should be inspected. (By the way, make sure everyone in your home knows where they are and if they are old enough, how to use them).—remember **PASS**? **P**ull–**A**im–**S**queeze–**S**weep.

3. What type of fire extinguishers to have, how many to have, and where to put them is also important. There is a lot of information on various online sites to help guide you. It is well worth a little research. Most recommend the Class ABC extinguishers as routine, at least one per floor and garage and basement. (A good idea would be to look at how far you would have to go to get to one. Class K or one that says 'for grease fires' should be in the kitchen).

4. How are you going to get out if you do have to evacuate?—you are laughing now because you think I am going to recommend having a fire drill once in a while. (I dare you guys to have it at six o'clock in the morning on your wife's day off—talk about fire…). Everyone should at least know how to evacuate with the fire being in different areas of the house. For example: if it's in the kitchen, follow *this* path. If it's coming from the basement or the dryer or wherever, have a planned exit.

5. If you have a two-story house and you can't get downstairs and out, make sure you what your exit plan is. I am hoping you say you have a rope ladder upstairs so you can use the lowest window to get everyone out. If you do not, get one, or at least have a solid plan to get out. (If there is any height to your house at all, jumping should not be considered an option).

We could certainly spend a lot more time on fires. Please do some additional research and see what you can do to keep your home safe from fires and make sure you and your family are prepared in case one occurs.

Other Safety Items in the Home

Again, volumes could be written here on the many things we could look at. The most common injuries are due to slips, trips, and falls. As I mentioned earlier, much of preventive health and safety can be taken care of by using your common sense. You don't need to hire a detective to find the things which may be safety or health issues. Just use your common sense.

Now watch as this old but speedy writer knocks a bunch out in record time.

1. The porch and side walk are icy——Scrape and put some salt down.
2. One of the sidewalk slabs is elevated——Level it out.
3. The basement floor is always damp and slippery— Get a dehumidifier.
4. The bathtub/shower is slippery ——Get a mat or some non-slip stickers.
5. The stair railing is loose——(Really?) Tighten it.
6. When I get up at night, I can't see in the hallway—— Get some little night lights.
7. I am so afraid one of the kids will get hurt in our automatic garage door——Keep the doors to the garage locked and never allow children in the garage unattended.
8. What about the pool?——Install a good security fence.
9. If you have coal, gas, oil, or wood heating——Don't forget about the Carbon Monoxide detectors. You should have one on every floor.

10. I am afraid my wife is going to…Set several reminders so that you don't forget your anniversary, AGAIN! (*An Ounce of Prevention*… Ha ha!).

Seriously, this is a rather lengthy book on Preventive Health and Safety. It could have saved many accidents and illnesses from occurring with just one phrase; *use common sense* and *stop, pause, and think* about what you are doing.

Earlier, I talked about a certain feeling you get when you are doing something that has a bit of a risk. Don't ignore it. Use it to employ some safety measures. On a roof, on a ladder, using a chainsaw, working with electricity, whatever it may be, just be extra careful and *think* before you *do*.

You could lose an eye weed eating if you don't have safety goggles on. Carelessness with a chainsaw could be very dangerous. Shut that breaker off before working on an electrical outlet. Consider scaffolding if you find yourself reaching a lot on the ladder. Always think of the worst possible scenario and compare it to just a little preventive measure, and you will do the right thing.

"Oh, darn, I forgot to get my goggles out of the garage. I don't feel like going way back over there to get them."

How would you feel about a glass eye then? See—no pun intended—what I mean. It's a no brainer.

The last general statement is difficult to put into words without being offensive. I want to say, *"Just don't do stupid stuff."* But that would not be very nice. So, I will stick with *Stop, Pause, and Think*.

I was working the ER one day and a man came in with burns all over his hands and arms. He was having a few beers while he was barbequing. Impatient with the coals not lighting, he decided to squirt some more lighter fuel in and had the bottle a bit too close to the fire—yep, you got it. I changed his dressings and debrided his burns every day for over a week.

Don't reach in to get your ring out of the garbage disposal until it is unplugged. But it's off, it should be OK— yes, Sally Seven Fingers said that too. I don't need a ladder, this folding chair will work—ya, go ahead, I am sure it will.

I also had a guy come into the Medical Aid Station one day who had a knife wound in his leg. He and a friend were playing some type of knife-dare game and his friend's knife slipped as he was throwing it, and well, I guess his friend was disqualified. Seven stitches later, this valiant winner claimed victory. Now I am not calling these people stupid but what they did was—ah, well not the best idea. I am sure you can think of several more. Just think and be safe. (Read the Appendix at the end. You may be able to relate to a few).

Chapter 12

Automobile Safety

Entire books have been written on this subject and I recommend you read some of them too—after you get all my books, of course. I love free advertising. I hate to keep repeating myself, but wow, traffic safety is a prime example of how common sense can prevent so many accidents. By the way, to show you just how serious this is, the National Highway Traffic Safety Administration says that there are about 5.5 million auto accidents each year, leading to over 3 million injuries and over 40,000 fatalities. (Can I please have your undivided attention for this section?)

As we look at this very important topic, we will look at both how to lower your risk of getting into an accident and also how to increase your odds of survival if you do happen to get into one. (Notice I said we will look at how to *lower your risk* of getting into an accident). There is no one hundred percent foolproof-method to prevent all accidents. I mentioned in the beginning, with other drivers involved, driving an automobile is always a risk.

Let's start with the car itself. Scott walks into the kitchen with a huge smile on his face.

"Hey honey!" he says to his wife. "Hello, what are you smiling about?"

"I just got the car inspected. I knew it wouldn't pass so I took it over to Al's garage. He passes everything. I was only in there five minutes. They call him lick 'em and stick 'em Al.

"Oh honey, I am so proud of you getting that done today; and without spending any money on silly repairs. Now, when I am on slippery surfaces, those bald tires will just help me slide right off the road. And those bad brakes won't stop on a dime, but they will stop when I hit that tree. You are just so smart." (You should have read this book first, Scott).

Please make sure your vehicles are in good shape. Sometimes there are horrible driving conditions due to weather and other events. Automobiles have to be in good condition in order to perform well driving defensively. Sometimes quick stops and turns are needed.

Here is a good one; *"Sometimes you should just not get into the car."*

"Well, then you won't go anywhere."

And I answer back, *"It's better not to go somewhere then it is to try and go somewhere if you have an increased risk of getting into an accident."*

If you have been drinking, do not drive that car; let someone that has not been drinking drive or just get a ride home.

Betty wakes up one morning and looks out the window. The car is parked half on the driveway and half in the yard. Fuming mad, she woke up her husband Hank.

"Hank, look at the way the car is parked. Did you drive home drunk last night?"

Hank was a bit groggy but answered, "No, I was smart. I asked Kevin to drive me home."

"Well then, how did the car get parked like that?" "Well, he was drunk too."

"Ha ha, yes Hank, you certainly were smart."

I just cannot stress enough on how important it is to grasp this fact: even if you don't think you are impaired or drunk, and you feel well enough to drive; please don't. According to the Center for Disease Control (CDC), there are over 10,800 fatalities a year due to drunk drivers. Over 1000 of these were children. Alcohol intoxicated drivers also cause over 290,000 injuries.

Personally, I would never risk all the trouble I would be in if I got a DUI, but so much more importantly, what if I would wreck? What if I would wreck into someone else? What if I killed someone, and perhaps a child or a baby? Could you live with any of that?—I know I couldn't. Trust me, it is never worth it. So, don't drink and drive.

I care about the people you may hurt if you cause an accident, but I also care about you. It's your life, and I don't think you want to go out early because you drank and drove. I doubt you want to spend the rest of your life paralyzed, or in a coma, or in a vegetative state, or permanently crippled, or even in prison. Hey, life is too fun to risk losing it all on a stupid decision to drive while you are under the influence. (Did I say stupid? I meant "a poor decision".......or did I???).

The same goes for anything that would impair your ability to drive responsibly, drive defensively, drive alertly, and drive safely. Let me know which of the drivers below should drive:

Angie: Just had knee surgery a few days ago but wants to go to her office. She pops a couple prescription pain pills and takes off in her car.

Kirk and Willie: They are partying with some street drugs and were asked to get more drinks. They get in the car and away they go.

Tommy: He works nights, but he stayed up and worked on the house all day. Now it's time for his forty-five-minute drive to work. Despite all the coffee he drank, he can barely keep his eyes open.

Melissa: She is having a migraine and has a bad headache, is nauseated, dizzy and lights hurt her eyes. The sun is just going down as she leaves work for her thirty-minute trip home.

Now if you said that none of these folks should be on the road, you are correct. They all have different reasons, but none of them should be behind the wheel. Avoiding the drive because of reasons like that may be inconvenient and the alternatives may require a little effort but it is certainly better than getting injured, injuring someone else, or worse. Remember, weigh the prevention against the worst-case scenario.

Now we are in the car. Everyone should be properly secured. There are laws for specific ages when restraining children. For example, in Virginia:

1. Infants must ride in the back seat in a rear facing safety child car seat. This should be done until the child is two years old or has outgrown the rear facing car seat.
2. Toddlers should ride in face forward car seat in the back seat with the five-point harness.
3. Children must ride in a car seat until they are eight years old. It may seem silly, but even children over eight who are not around 4'9" should also continue to ride in the booster seat. Remember, the concept here is for the regular seatbelt to fit the child properly. Many times, in shorter children, the shoulder strap lies close to the neck. Not good placement.
4. Adults, buckle up, and buckle up properly. Wearing seatbelts improperly can also be very dangerous.

"Ha, I hate that annoying sound when I am not wearing my seatbelt, so I went under the seat and disconnected it," "Well, I just keep the seatbelt buckled behind me." Good thinking. You have just negated a preventive measure which has saved thousands of

lives. I just hope you don't regret it. (If you get in an accident…for sure you will).

Now let's talk about my favorite topic, driving distracted. When you are driving a motor vehicle at any speed at all, you are encountering a risk. The things you do while you are driving and the way you drive will determine how big of a risk it actually is. Taking your eyes off of the road, even for a short time, could cause a serious accident. How long does it take to swerve out of your lane or off the road? It takes very little time and less as your speed increases. Even at thirty-five to forty- five miles per hour, you and the other people involved can be seriously injured or killed. When you are not focused on the road, you can miss seeing pedestrians, vehicles passing you, vehicles pulling out of driveways, and the ever so popular, vehicles slowing quickly or stopping in front of you.

Please take the time to think about the possible end results of being distracted with something else in the car. How would you live the rest of your life knowing that what you were doing ended up causing an accident which took the life of a passenger in your car, perhaps one of your children or a spouse? It would be a solemn regret that would follow you all your life. Or how about the accident causing you or someone in another vehicle to be paralyzed or perhaps lose a limb, or an eye? As I am writing this, there are many people in comas who were victims of a car accident which was caused by another driver, driving distracted. Yes, I wanted it to look as horrible as I can make it because it happens all the time.

So, what are some of the distractions? It can be absolutely anything. Eating, daydreaming, kids misbehaving, and cell phones are just to name a few. Cell phones have been such a huge technological advancement, sometimes I wonder how we ever lived without them. But they can cause serious trouble in the car. Many states are requiring hands free telephone use for that very reason.

Here is Brenda. She just broke up with her boyfriend at a party and is a bit teary eyed. She was with her girlfriends, and they were all trying to console her. She left the party to drive home. Soon she started getting texts from all her girlfriends. She quickly answered one and just as she hit *Send*, she heard a noise. She ran over the rumble strips. It startled her a bit, so she laid her phone down in the car.

NOTE: (Please read this carefully) If you know texting and driving is dangerous, *please don't text someone who is driving*. Only makes sense, right?

She decided not to read the texts, but she did look to see who they were from. Then it happened, a text came in from her ex-boyfriend. When she saw it, she forgot all about the rumble strips and couldn't wait to see if he was sorry and wanted to get back together. She opened it, took a look at the road, and then started reading the text.

Suddenly, she heard another noise. It wasn't the rumble strips this time, it was a pickup truck horn blowing. She had swerved into the other lane and was heading straight into the path of the truck—OK, let's stop there. I think you get the picture.

I was not always the safe, model driver that I am today. (Please don't ask my daughter about the validity of that last statement). My big problem was that I loved to look around while I drove. I looked for deer, pretty scenery, just about anything, so I did have to do some lane adjustments once and a while. I live close to Goshen Pass in Virginia. It is so beautiful, but the roads are narrow and a bit difficult to navigate if you are looking at the beautiful river. Keep your eyes on the road.

Long drives are the worst, although if you mess around in the car, it doesn't matter how far you go. Long drives make me want to check emails, texts, the news, anything to pass the time. If you are like that, try getting some good audio books that you can really get into. Whatever you do, stay alert, don't do things that will take your eyes and attention from driving. Believe me, the risk is high enough each time you venture out in that vehicle, you don't need to make it any worse.

It is really scary driving down the road and have someone pass you, (My daughter would also tell you that everyone passes me. What's with her, right?) and they have both hands on something besides the steering wheel. Food, phones, iPads, cigarette and lighter, make up brushes, and eye liners. Some have that visor mirror down looking at themselves in it. *Get up earlier and get ready before you get into the car.*

Then there are the people who have to look at each other while they are driving. I have seen some good fights in moving vehicles going at least sixty miles per hour, I'll never know how they do it. Some people get the edge arguing with that LOOK. (You know what I am talking about guys. Now, I didn't say ladies do it, I was just asking… ah, never mind). Keep your eyes on the road. They can hear you without you looking at them.

If the kids are misbehaving in the back seat, don't turn around to see what they are doing. Pull over when it is safe to check it out. Taking your eyes off the road is extremely dangerous, even for just a few seconds. Sometimes, safety takes time. It's better to spend time being safe than saving time and having a tragedy come your way.

I could write and write and write about automobile safety. Just use caution, common sense, and always think that if you don't, you might not get to where you are going. So, let's wrap this up with a few other items.

1. Speed limits are in place for a reason. The slower the limit, the more dangerous the area is. *"The speed limit here is 25mph. The road is fine."* And so are all the little children who live close to that road.

2. Yellow lights mean slow down and prepare to stop, not *"gun it and beat the red light."*
3. Yield means ah, well, *to yield.* The other drivers have the right of way, and you are to yield it to them.
4. Slow down when there are poor road conditions.
5. Driving a vehicle is not the time or place to show how brave you are or how silly you can be—hey, I was a teenager, once upon a time, far, far away. It seems cool. Guess what, so is the morgue. Each year, over 5,000 young people (Sixteen to twenty years old) die in automobile accidents. Over 400,000 are seriously injured.

NOTE: There is a section in the front of my senior high school yearbook that has a *Dedication* section. Four of the pictures in that section were of guys on my baseball team. They were all killed in the same car accident.

6. Anytime you see something that could pose a danger, slow down. Bad roads, children playing, a vehicle on the other side of the road, and other pedestrians.
7. If you are drowsy, pull over, get some rest or something to munch on and drink. Walk around a bit but never drive drowsy. You can and will fall asleep without ever knowing it and may never wake up.

You saw the statistics. You don't want to take a chance on killing or hurting yourself or others.

NOTE ON RUSHING: You can rush doing many things and not increase your risk of an injury, but driving is not one of them.

See if you recognize any of those actions that are often done when rushing while behind the wheel:

1. The windshield is still frosty but you keep wiping it and using your windshield washer and wipers so you can see out a little clearing.
2. You hit the gas at all the yellow lights to beat the red light. Sometimes you do, sometimes you don't.
3. You make quick lane changes to get around slower vehicles and pass in "no passing" zones.
4. You totally ignore yield signs.
5. You maintain your speed through construction areas and in bad driving conditions.
6. You become a very agitated and uncourteous driver.
7. You drive way too fast and well over the speed limit.
8. You wait until the last minute to get into the slower turning lane to make a turn and usually cut in front of someone to get over.
9. You do not come to a complete stop at "Stop" signs.

Any of these sound familiar? Get up *earlier*, leave *earlier*, allow yourself *more* time; and drive *safely*. And if for some reason you are still going to be late, remember that it is better to get to your destination a little later than to get to a hospital in the back of a speeding ambulance.

Chapter 13

Enduring Illness or Enjoying Wellness

Wellness is being in a state of good health. I wish our actions could ensure wellness, but even with the best attempts at remaining healthy, people still develop serious illnesses and medical conditions. You have probably heard stories of people who ate right, exercised regularly, and did everything they were supposed to do to be healthy, but die young from a massive heart attack. Or perhaps someone who has never smoked developing lung cancer at an early age. Yes, these situations do happen, but the statistics prove that you have a much higher chance of avoiding conditions like that if you practice a healthy lifestyle.

I have recommended this in almost every section of this book, but particularly here I implore you to do some reading and research on the topic of wellness. We are going to talk a bit about diet, exercise, and basic wellness practices. There are also so many good books out there, along with articles on the internet to give you much more detailed information, so we will just skim the surface.

As we have been discussing in prevention, you have to have the right mindset if you really want to take this seriously.

Ignoring the need or belittling the benefits of healthy living can land you in deep trouble. It is also a matter of 'now vs later.' (See more details in my book, *Successfully Programming Your Mind*). What you do now will affect how you fare in the future. Is having a ball in your twenties, thirties, and forties worth enduring health conditions, surgeries, strokes, heart attacks, or cancer in your fifties, sixties, and seventies?

In my first book, *Reincarnate Now*, I talk about the millions of people who live with deep regrets over mistakes they made in the past. Some of those were over neglecting their health. A woman who smoked all her life has developed lung cancer. She has a life expectance of only a few months and will most likely not live long enough to see her first grandchild born.

A man who hardly ever exercised and since about thirty years old, had been way over his ideal weight, had a stroke at fifty-seven years old. He is still slightly paralyzed on his left side, unable to speak, and can't walk or use his left arm.

Here is another one with an almost identical story as the last one but she died of a massive heart attack at fifty-nine years old.

Now, what do all these people have in common? They would all have wished that they could go back in time and live a healthier life. Some of you who are inflicted with a serious illness are nodding your head and saying, *"I know I sure wish I could."* Some of you younger healthy people who are starting out as they did are saying, *"Well, that won't happen to me."*

I have to tell this story and you may have already heard it. I think it illustrates what I am saying but if not, I still enjoy telling it.

The dam was about to break above a small town. The occupants were being evacuated. When the police got to one old man's house, the old man said, *"You all go on, God will take care of me."* The waters started to rise and the man climbed up on his porch roof. A rescue boat came by to get him but he repeated, *"You all go on, God will take care of me."* Finally, the water came barreling down and the man crawled up on his house top. A rescue helicopter came by to get him and yet again he said, *"You all go on, God will take care of me."* The man was swept away and drowned. When he got to heaven, he said to the Lord, *"I trusted you God and I died in that flood."* The Lord said, *"I sent a car, a boat, and a helicopter to get you, what more could I do?"* (I can hear the roars of laughter).

That is why people in the medical field get so frustrated. We try so hard to warn people, just like the American Heart Association, and the American Cancer Society, and others, but people say, *"You all go on, I'll be fine."* Please, I beg you, take this seriously and start immediately. The longer you wait to start healthy living the more opportunity you are giving disease processes to start working against you.

One more comment and we will get started—man, this was a longer introduction on this section than I thought it was going to be, must be important huh???

As a parent, one of the best things you can do is to get your children started on the right foot and instill in them how important it is to develop and maintain a healthy lifestyle. It will take persistence and consistent messaging, but it will be worth it. But believe me, it won't be easy.

In case you haven't noticed, our nation has a tremendous obesity problem. It stems from our next two topics, diet, and exercise. Some of our problems are due to the lifestyles we live. Most families now have two working parents, so that often means, fast food time, and what child minds that?—*"But daddy, there are no green, leafy vegetables in my happy meal."* And since both parents are tired from work, the fun in the back yard has turned into TV and video games.

Chapter 14

What You Are Eating May Be Eating You!

I am not a dietitian or a nutritionist, so I will be sticking to very general guidelines. (Please look up some references on the internet). There are also a ton of good books on nutrition. It may be good to ask your doctor for a nutritional consult as well. With everything that is available, there is no excuse for not knowing how to eat healthy foods.

Since I am writing this book and such a model example, I was going to just give you a list of all the foods that I mostly ate as a young and middle-aged adult. Then tell you to avoid all the foods on the list. I have to admit, I have an *'I'* problem. (Spaghetti, Rigatoni, Linguini, Stromboli, Ravioli), I would probably eat a cardboard box if it had spaghetti sauce on it. I just love pasta—I told you, I had quadruple bypass surgery. The inside of my arteries probably looked like a garbage disposal at an Italian restaurant.

OK, back to you, I spanked me long enough. I think our bodies start out very young saying, *"Put that yucky good stuff away and bring on the goooood stuff."* OK, moms, think back. The baby is in the highchair and it's feeding time. (Oh, sorry, that sounded terrible like at the zoo). It's time to feed the baby. (That's better). You have a jar of green beans and a jar of applesauce or pears. Which is easier to get them to eat?

I used to trick my kids. I'd give them a spoon of applesauce and then another and then a spoonful of green beans or carrots. It would usually end up on the bib after they would make a really mean face at me. Face it, kids will want the good stuff over the healthy stuff every time.

One more story—yes, you should know by now, I tell a lot of stories. When my brother and I were young, we lived on top of a lane. My grandma, aunt, and uncle lived at the bottom, right across from the bus stop. When we got off, grandma would always be on the porch. *"Hey boys, come and see grandma."* She would always ask us the same question, *"You boys want a couple cookies and some milk?"* She would tell us not to eat too many so we would still be hungry for supper, but we would dunk those Oreos in milk till our fingers were wrinkled. You are not going to believe this… we were not hungry for supper. It will be hard, it will be a fight, it will make you feel bad at times, but if you can get them into a habit of eating right, you may just prevent an early death or serious health condition.

Here is a dietary thought: divide your plate into four sections. Half of the plate should be taken up with fruits and vegetables, (except potatoes). One forth with whole grains, (PASTA yeah!!! But the whole wheat type, oh…). And one forth with protein, (non-red meats are preferred.) Avoid processed meats like bacon or sausage. *"I love cheap BOLOGNA, and I cannot lie; if I don't stop eating it, I'm surely gonna die."* (Yes, I am a song writer too).

Now, I want to make a statement that I want you to read very carefully. After you do your research to see what you can eat and what you should avoid, use that information as a guide to construct eating and meal planning habits. This is one area that I say: just do the best you can.

So how can we gage how we are doing? First of all, there is your weight. There are plenty of charts that will tell you what your ideal body should be. I am right at my ideal body weight at sixty-five years old—if I was 7'6" tall. Ha ha. Just kidding, a bit. Then there is your Body Mass Index, (BMI), which looks at the relationship between your weight and your height. In adults, a Body Mass Index of 25 or more is considered overweight. Over 30, then, would be defined as obese. Ask your MD during your next visit where you stand or look up BMI calculators online. The calculation is simply multiplying your weight by 703, and then dividing it by your height in inches twice. So, if a person is six foot tall and weighs a hundred and eight pounds, it would calculate like this: (180 X 703) / 72 / 72 = 24.4%. Looking good!

Just a few more things on diet and that will be it. It's nearly time for my apple pie and ice cream. (Ha ha! I wish.)

1. Portion control. Don't let how good everything tastes determine how much you are going to eat. Determine that as you fix your plate and stick to it.
2. Watch the subconscious grazing. I did it all the time. I try to use portion control at meal times to cut down on calories, then I grab a bite of this here, finish the little bite out of this bowl (Can't put just two bites away and who wants to waste good food, right?), grab some chips, eat a cookie. Well guess what, I just defeated the purpose for watching my portions.
3. Drink six to eight glasses of water a day.
4. Eat slowly! It has been proved that the mind is a bit slow to register you are full. Ever eat so much you feel like you are going to explode, especially around the holidays? Your mind fails to report to your mouth that you are full and so you just keep on going.

5. AVOID crash diets. This is not a sprint, it's a marathon. (For me, it has been several marathons). You want consistent lifestyle changes instead of most of the fad, *Gone But It's Back Again* diets. (Also named: *The Room Spins When I Stand Up* diets). They are unhealthy and most of them are unsustainable.

6. Be reasonable and patient. Eat right, exercise, and follow your doctor or nutritionist's recommendation for a healthy diet. You will find that you will progress gradually, and it will be a permanent change.

7. Be sensible. Many people die each year from eating disorders developed by trying to be skinny. (See my book, *It's Not **What** Things You See; It's **How** You See Things*). You are not trying to look like a model or actor or actress on TV. The real you is inside. Now for health purposes, get in the best shape you can, but please don't compare yourself with Hollywood.

NOTE: *Please remember to talk to your physician about a diet which fits your health needs, especially those of you who have chronic conditions like diabetes and kidney failure. Many of the things discussed above may not fit into your particular nutritional plan.*

Chapter 15

Exercise

Oh, boy, we finally arrived at my favorite topic. Starting an exercise program is one of the easiest things to do. I have done it a hundred times. But keeping up with an exercise program? Now why did you have to go and ask that? Like dieting, exercise should have a few guidelines. Exercise too, should be a gradual process. I am not talking about preparing to try out for Mr. or Mrs. Universe, I am talking about a good exercise program which gets your heart beating, your lungs breathing, and stressing your muscles a bit.

The key here is consistency. You really have to be determined to keep an exercise program up. Guess the answers to these questions:

1. What is the top enrollment month for fitness centers and gyms?
2. When are the fitness centers and gyms back to their usual customers?
3. How many months does it take for the treadmill, exercise bike, and weight station to accumulate dust?
4. How many days a year is it not too hot, not too cold, and not to wet to take a nice walk? (Oh, and not too buggy).

I think you know what I am getting at. We have talked a lot about prevention. Preventing serious health conditions is worth the effort believe me. The people who are living through that right now would tell you that if they could, they would go back and take better care of their bodies. Then there are those who can't tell you anything because they did not live through the heart attack, or stroke, or other fatal medical condition.

Here you are, it's a Tuesday night and you started an exercise program where you walk on the treadmill—it's too cold outside—for two miles and spend thirty minutes lifting weights, every other day. It's winter, so it is dark by time you get home from your very hectic day. It's seven o'clock in the evening, and you just got done eating and doing dishes. (Did I tell you guys that helping with the dishes is a way to prevent an injury? Ha ha).

So, you are beat, and that recliner sure looks good. Would it hurt if he just took a night off? Absolutely not, BUT, you know it will turn into two nights next week, then three, then a whole week off, but then he starts back strong, and then quits altogether. Like dieting, an exercise program is very hard to keep up.

There are tons of articles, books, and resources to guide you on your exercise journey, so I am not going to go into great detail.

Just a few things on the more practical side:

1. It is always best to see your doctor before you start a rigorous exercise program. If you are in your mature years—what a nice way to put that—you should discuss any exercise program with your doctor. Moderate paced walking in moderation is usually pretty well tolerated but better safe than sorry. (You need a check-up anyhow).

2. As I mentioned, take it slow and build yourself up gradually. *"My first bike ride in twenty years, let's see if we can make ten miles."* You may want to start out on a bit shorter goal there, Chipper. Muscles like exercise and they like to grow and expand, but they like to do it slowly. They also like twenty hours between workouts to recover and mend.

3. If you men want to "woo" the girls or vice versa, lift for bulk. The rest of us, lift for tone. Less weight and more reps will help get those muscles in good shape. I have to tell this story: I have never seen someone laugh to the point of tears in a gym. I signed up for a gym membership in January. (Oh crap, gave away one of the answers to the quiz I gave you.) There was a quasi-trainer walking around helping everyone. He asked me if I was looking to add bulk or just to tone up. I looked as serious as I could and said, *"I don't think I can bulk up much more. I'm already having trouble finding shirts that will fit."* I thought he was going to die laughing. Hey, now that I think about it, that wasn't very nice. That's probably why I quit in March. (Ohhh, there goes another answer…).

4. It is good to try and make your exercise time as fun as possible. When you can walk outside, find a good place to walk where you can enjoy the scenery. When on the treadmill or lifting, put something on to listen to, like music or a book, or some podcasts. I always put a mix of all the Rocky theme songs. The last little bit, I crank up that speed and lift the incline and there I go up those steps… Da da da……. Da da da. Then I collapse on the nearby couch and pant for twenty minutes.

5. Do not compare yourself with others. You are working on you to become the best version of you. Don't worry

about Mr. Abs next door or Mrs.-Size-Minus-Two down the block. Just be a good, healthy you!

6. Make sure you stay hydrated. Some people think when they see all the perspiration, *"Boy, I am losing weight now."* Ah, that would be water, not fat. Losing too much water too fast could make your blood pressure drop.

7. Slow and steady sails the exercise ship into fitness. Many people start fast and furious and end up quitting.

8. Again, be more concerned about how you feel instead of how you look. Your health and longevity of life provide far better motivation than popularity and turning heads.

Chapter 16

Preventive Healthcare and Screenings

This is another really important and possibly life-saving chapter. I want you to do yourself a favor and get with your doctor to create a preventive healthcare plan for you. Some people need to see the doctor more often, so I don't really give blanket guidelines but suggestions to at least get you started.

In starting, I want to make a few general comments. Our nation is in a healthcare crisis both in staffing and in finances. Both of these issues would be helped if we had a huge increase in preventive healthcare participants. (For example: what do you think will cost more? A colonoscopy at fifty years old, or a massive colon resection surgery, colostomy creation, cancer therapy, etc.?)… I think you get the idea. Early detection and prevention are key.

Accidents are not the only thing we can prevent. There are many serious and fatal health conditions we can prevent or at least catch in time to effectively treat. We will discuss specific measures a bit later but let's lay some foundations.

Rate yourself on this scale. How important is preventive healthcare to you?

4 – *Very Important*
3 – *Somewhat Important*
2 – *Not really important*
1 – *Not important*

Now, did you answer according to what you think or how you participate? If you rated yourself a **4** but have not had all your recommended vaccines, screenings, or had at least an annual check-up, then you think it is very important, but you do not translate that belief into action. If I am drowning and someone throws me a life preserver, I can believe all I want that it can save me, but if I don't grab it, I will sink. (Personally, I can't float a lick. I jump in and swim. If I stop, I go straight to the bottom. A lot of muscle mass must do that, you think? [insert smiley face]).

Here is our friend Lewis. He is one of those rough and tough guys. He has never called in sick, never been in a hospital as a patient and never felt the need to see a doctor. He has headaches sometimes, but doesn't everyone? Probably just sinuses he would say. He is sixty-seven years old and just about to retire when his symptoms hit. When he finally saw a doctor, his blood pressure was high. Undoubtedly, it had been high for years. The doctor asked him if it had ever been high before and he said, *"Don't know, never had it checked."* Lewis now is spending his much-deserved retirement on dialysis. If I had a dime for every patient who matched that scenario, I could retire. It happens a lot. Now wouldn't it have been much easier to have had some preventive health check-ups along the way and avoided renal failure?

One of the goals of P.H.A.S.E. is to help people realize how important preventive healthcare is. That includes screenings, vaccines, checkups, and many other things. I guarantee that if dialysis patients could travel back in time, they would have taken preventive healthcare more seriously.

Do you know through preventive measures, we have eradicated several diseases? Vaccines are preventive measures which prevent someone from getting a particular disease. Say goodbye to polio, tetanus, rubella, and more. All because we found ways to prevent them. What did you say there, sir? *"I'm not taking the flu shot. I don't need that pneumonia shot. Doc says I should get a Shingles vaccine, but I had the chicken pox, so I don't need it."* Well, if you don't take the vaccine to PREVENT those diseases, you may very well get them. That is what prevention is all about. (By the way, look at the statistics on how many people, especially the elderly and people with other medical conditions, die each year from pneumonia and the flu). And anyone who has had shingles will tell you that they wished they had taken the vaccine. It is extremely painful.

Andy and Cheryl are camping. They had such a nice fire going but it was time to leave. Andy poured water on the fire. Then he stirred it around a bit and poured more water on it. Then he covered it all with dirt and threw more water on it. (You say: *man that guy is a bit off. He is really over doing it).* No, he is *PREVENTING* a forest fire. (Remember Smokey the Bear? Not Yogi). Think that was excessive? Ask the firefighters in California if they think it was excessive. Doing what Andy did can prevent thousands of acres and hundreds of homes from catching fire. Thanks Andy, you are the man! (You must be asking what that has to do with healthcare? I have no idea, but it was cool right?). The concept is as the title of the book states, (Now you are saying, ya, what was the title of this book?). An ounce of prevention is worth a lot more than you can imagine.

Barry is laughing at Dave because he slobbered a bit while drinking some water. Dave just got back from the dentist and his mouth was still a bit numb. *"I've never had a filling. That is just one of the ways that dentist make money. You have a cavity that needs filled. That will be two-hundred and fifty dollars."* Dave told him that their insurance covered most of it and they also paid for exams and cleanings. (Remind me to come back to that point). Barry was eating popcorn that night and caught a kernel in the wrong place and—hey, don't jump ahead. Let me tell the story—*crack!* he broke a tooth. Now he had to go to the dentist. Come to find out, his tooth was infected and abscessed. He ended up having to have a root canal and a crown put on, that cost him a pretty penny. Guess what the dentist told him… go ahead guess? Yep, you're right: *"If you would have had this cavity filled a while back, we wouldn't have had to do all of this. You have eight other cavities. Do you want to schedule your next visit so we can get started on them?"*

"Yu wa shh ru geee aaaha beerrr nunnn." was Barry's response with a suction, two other instruments, and three fingers in his mouth. (Did you ever notice that the dentist shoves a bunch of stuff in your mouth and then starts a conversation? Funny thing is, they understand every word you say).

"Great sir, yes we have some late afternoon appointments." Ha ha, go figure.

Now what did I tell you to remind me of? Oh yes, did you ever wonder why insurance companies give you free dental exams and cleanings and free physicals? Because they are *preventive.* They can help identify things that could turn into serious conditions later on down the road and cost them a lot and cost you your health or life. Now they have nurses calling to check on you, dietitians available to help with nutritional counselling, and even talk lines for depression and stress. Why? Because they know the value of prevention and early detection.

Tom is a hard-working guy who loves his job even though it is very stressful at times, he loves his family and loves to EAT. Tom is very overweight, has high cholesterol, and high blood pressure. Basically, he is a model example of what a high-risk candidate for cardiac disease looks like. So now I want you to get this: *Sometimes the ounce of prevention isn't easy; but it is still an ounce compared to the alternative.* His doctor gave him a diet to follow, a weight loss plan, an exercise regimen, and some blood pressure medications to take. Guess what wasn't on his diet plan that was on the menu at his favorite Italian restaurant? Almost everything. So now it is not going to be easy, but I PERSONALLY guarantee it will be worth it.

Tom and I have a lot in common. Back in 2009, I was having some heart problems, so I had a stress test. I failed that so they set me up for a cardiac catherization. I woke up at the end and could see my heart on the TV screen. I said, *"Hey, that looks pretty normal to me."*

The Cardiologist said, *"Far from it my friend."*

"Oh, well what do I know, I am all drugged up." The Doc had to laugh but my results were not funny. To make a long story short, two weeks later I had quadruple bypass surgery, recovered well and the entire time I was wishing that I would have never gotten to that point. Prevention would have been sweeeeeet. (Did you know that they make some spaghetti noodles out of squash? Mmmmm, yummy!). So, trust me, if you can prevent heart conditions and avoid open heart surgery, do it!

Polly is forty-five years old and in great health. She is a sun lover and lives for summertime and the beach, and she still looks pretty good in a bikini. (No honey, I wasn't staring at her. She is a character in the book, so stop looking over my shoulder while I am writing). She loved to tan so used the lower SPF sunscreen. She would visit her mother who would always comment on how tanned she was and with her silky, blonde hair, she looked like a model. One day after playing racquetball, she was getting dressed in the locker room when another lady walked by.

"Excuse me, I am not snooping or anything, but I am a nurse and noticed that you have a few dark spots in the middle of your back. One of them looks kind of suspicious. You should have it checked."

"Thanks, I will."

Well, she strained to see the spots in the mirror, and they looked fine to her. She did remember that her best friend knew someone who had to have a melanoma removed and the doctor told her that those who stay out in the sun a lot and don't protect their skin should have periodic skin cancer screenings. Well, she didn't go for a screening and two years later... well, let's just say, an ounce of prevention would have been much better.

So, let's look at a few suggestions on screenings and vaccines.

1. *Well Baby Checks*: Many children develop conditions because they do not have regular checkups in infancy. Recommendations are that babies should be seen by a pediatrician at one, two, four, six, nine, twelve, fifteen, eighteen, and twenty-four months old. (American Academy of Pediatrics). You may think that is a lot, but they don't need their tires rotated every visit. (Joke there, just a joke...).

2. *Infant Immunizations*: If you follow the well-baby exam schedule above, the pediatric clinic will make sure your child gets their needed immunizations. Any pediatric clinic will have handouts on the scheduled vaccines. Don't miss them or take them lightly. Many diseases have been totally irradicated by having these vaccines administered down through the years.

3. *Annual Exams:* These should be done, ah, well, annually. If you notice, most insurance companies pay for one annual exam. They realize how important these exams are for early detection of conditions that could lead to serious illnesses.

4. *General Recommended Screenings:* As I have mentioned several times, do your research on all these screenings. Family history and your medical history can have a lot to do with when the screenings should start and how

often they should be done. But as a general guideline some of the screenings include:

a. Cholesterol

b. Skin exams for suspicious moles or skin lesions

c. Breast exams and mammograms. Mammograms usually are started at around age forty years old and are done annually.

d. Men's prostate screenings start at around fifty years old.

e. Colonoscopies usually start at fifty years old and are done every ten years if results are normal.

f. At around sixty-five years old, your physician may recommend a bone density study and continue to get them every few years.

g. Don't forget all the immunizations like the yearly flu shot, pneumonia, shingles, and any others recommended by your physician.

Chapter 17

Procrastination: Prevention and Safety Can't Wait!

The last point I make in my book, *Reincarnate Now,* is how dangerous and defeating procrastination is. Do you want to make changes in your life? Then start now. Do you want to quit smoking, start exercising, start dieting, make that career move, go back to school? Then get started right away. Do you want your family to be engaged in safety and preventive healthcare? Then start NOW!

Intentions are only good if they are acted upon quickly. My tires are getting slick, I am going to get new ones. My brakes are squealing, I am going to get them checked. I am going to put a fence up around the pool. I am going to check all the fire extinguishers and smoke alarms. I am going to change all the outlets to safety outlets. I am going to fix that loose step. I am going to have that colonoscopy done. I am going to get a mammogram and PAP smear done. I am going to have a dermatologist look at some of these spots that have come up.

All of these are good intentions, but they are USELESS unless they actually get done.

Andy was fifty years old. He was good and went in for his annual check-up. He smoked and had a chronic cough, so the doctor ordered an x-ray. It showed two small spots. He ordered a scan just to check it out but told Andy not to be alarmed yet as it might not be anything. The next day at work, an older co-worker told Andy that he had the same thing, had all the scans done and it was nothing, probably from smoking too long. Andy put the scan off and didn't think any more about it over the next year and a half. He started losing weight and feeling tired all the time. He went back in and finally had a scan done. It was cancer after all but it had now had spread. Andy was in for some rough days, as many as he had left.

Over the next several weeks, Andy kept asking himself, *"Why didn't I get that scan done years ago?"* He agreed that he needed it done and there was no reason not to get it done. He just procrastinated and it cost him. Now was that an actual story? No, just an example. But does this happen all the time, certainly. Many people INTEND to get things done but just don't do it.

How about some other possible stories? The fence never did get built and a toddler from next door stumbled and fell into the pool. The man with the bald tires was driving home in a bad storm and didn't make a sharp curve in the road. A house caught fire with all the family asleep inside, the smoke detector batteries had been dead for months. The sun-loving lady started to cry as the doctor told her that one of spots was a melanoma.

Again, just examples but I can't stress enough that these things happen all the time. When you procrastinate engaging preventive measures, you move from the lower risk area of prevention to the higher risk area of chance. When it comes to prevention, consciously pause, and think about it, decide what needs to be done and DO IT, and as quickly as possible.

Now you are stopping, PAUSING, (I hope), and thinking about some of the things you have read. The real question is, what are you going to DO? Not just think about doing, or intending to do, but taking action and doing it. Get that phone out and make a screening appointment. Start putting your seatbelt on. Change the batteries in the smoke detectors and make sure they are functioning. Just be fully engaged in prevention because, *An Ounce of Prevention Is Worth More Than You Can Imagine.*

One final story. During my career in the USAF, I was on the Honor Guard. One thing that we did was shoot the 21-gun salute at military funerals. We always got to the cemetery early and I usually wondered around a bit looking at headstones. That drove home a very valuable lesson. Death is no respecter of age. There were people buried who had died in their nineties but there were also middle-aged and young adults, teenagers, and yes, children and babies.

Now we all know that people do get sick and die. We hate it but it happens, but in any cemetery, I am sure there are those buried there who died pre-maturely due to a lack of either safety or preventive health measures. Some from accidents, and others from illnesses which may have been prevented by vaccines, screenings, or regular exams. You do not have to look through a cemetery to learn that lesson. I think you know it already. Now, what are you going to DO about it?

By the way, the first funeral I went to with the Honor Guard was for a man killed in a hunting accident. Someone saw some bushes moving and thought it was a deer; it wasn't.

Final thought: Safety and Preventive Health isn't just about not doing things wrong, it's also about starting to do things right. Want to sleep well at night and be confident that you and your loved ones will be OK? Where would you rather base your confidence, in the preventive measures that we just talked about or just CHANCE?

"I have those screenings, blood tests, and exams done all the time. They never find anything." That is great, and you really haven't lost everything and have gained a little assurance that you are in good health. The reverse question is, what will you lose if you do have something wrong and don't get it checked? Trust me now, it is not worth the risk. Be safe.... PHASE ON!

Chapter 18

An Ounce of Tips

We have looked at so many ways you can use prevention both with accidents and health issues. Here are just a few tips that can be helpful in being able ensure you use these preventive measures.

I have found, and I am sure you will agree, that reminders are a great way of helping you not forget things. People used to tie a string around their finger to remind them of something important. My problem would be, I would have to set another reminder to remind me of what the string was for. Nonetheless, they can be very useful.

A subtle reminder is good on the fridge or near the treats of your desire to eat healthier is a good example. As I mentioned earlier, sometimes we automatically do things without really stopping to think about what we are doing. We just subconsciously grab that little snack. Keep it positive though. Don't use signs like, *"If you eat that, you are going to stay fat."* Just a simple, *"I can do this,"* or *"The healthier me is coming"* will suffice. A habit of healthy eating takes time to develop so using reminders is a good way to help until you get there.

Sticking with eating tips, one huge problem I have is cooking too much. I used to just grab a huge handful of spaghetti and throw it in the pot. After my other half and I were done eating, there was a lot left over and BINGO, seconds. Now I use a measuring device to give us plenty for healthy portions and a little extra for her lunch the next day. And I eliminated the temptation to grab a second serving. We also do the same with another favorite, potatoes. Lots of extra potatoes in the pot cry out to me, *"Here I am, come and get me."* As you know, a little here and a little there and the little diet plan is out the window.

Bread with meals really adds a lot of extra carbs and fat also. We now have salads with our pasta meals and have cut back on several pieces of garlic bread. If we do have bread with meals, it is just one piece—a piece. (That sounds funny, one piece, a piece). Anyhow, it is a helpful practice.

I mentioned the one medication I had to start taking with my supper meal. How did I finally get that on autopilot? I set the medication bottle next to the place I have the dish drying towel hanging. So, each time I grabbed the towel, it served as a reminder so I never missed taking my medication. Now you say, *"What if you didn't dry dishes?"* Well, I would have a lot more health concerns than just missing the medication. *OUCH!!* (No, I am not hen-pecked, just considerate).

Safety reminders are also a good practice. Get into a habit of doing things that will increase the likelihood of using preventive measures and thus reducing your risk. Placing your safety goggles next to the weed eater or chainsaw is a great example. Calendar reminders are good for smoke detector and fire extinguisher checks. I have a drawer of electrical outlets and switches. I cut out a little lightning bolt picture and taped it to the drawer. It serves as a reminder to turn that breaker off first.

In the car, we need all the reminders we can get. P.H.A.S.E. will soon be giving out arm bracelets and other reminders. Put one in the car just to remind you that you are about to enter a very risky situation. Using good driving practices will help reduce the risk. I am sure you can think of reminders to make sure you don't forget the little one in the back seat. For one, put a pacifier on your door handle. When you touch it as you open your door, it will remind you to make sure you dropped the little tyke off at daycare.

Getting support is also so very important. Get your family, friends, and coworkers more concerned about safety and preventive healthcare. They can really be an encouragement as you try to diet, exercise, stop smoking, and incorporating other good preventive healthcare measures. Have them buy this book and… (Ha ha, more free advertising).

Here is a good example. My first lunch while working in the hospital ER was interrupted after five minutes for an emergency. Working in EMS, I cannot tell you how many calls we got just as we pulled out of the drive through. Conclusion: I developed a practice of eating very fast. I know, it's horrible but after all these years, it's really hard to break that routine.

Now my other half has a habit of phone-eating. She takes a bite and then says hi to twenty Facebook friends, answers two texts, and so on. Needless to say, I am done eating before she finishes her salad. I was going to try and only take a bite when she did but come on, I would starve, and the food gets cold. So, when I was done eating and she was just halfway done, what would I do? Sit there and peck and eat and eat and peck. Finally, we agreed that I would finish eating and excuse myself and wait an hour until she finished to start cleaning up. (P.S. This is just my personal opinion but if I could, I would ban phones from the dinner table. What happened to good family conversation time?). At any rate, it helped me stop grazing after I was done.

When someone who is trying to stop smoking says they really would love to have one, be that support for them. Find people to walk or exercise with. It will keep you both working toward that goal.

Right Way: "Hey honey, would you go for a walk with me. I am trying to get in better shape and it would be nice to walk together." (Ahhhh, nice touch.)

Wrong Way: "Hey honey, come walk with me. I am trying to get in better shape and you could shed a few pounds yourself." Are you mad?… I mean, your walk may have just turned into a sprint, and I bet she will catch you.

Whew! That was a scarry ending. Here is another thing that can help. Make sure you get your doctor visits scheduled and make a list of all the things you want to discuss with them. Don't stop until you covered your list. Is it time for a vaccine, flu shot, screenings needed? Discuss any things you may feel are important to your health. Sometimes they hurry and miss some relevant questions. Make a good list so you do not forget. Also ask about the labs you will be getting and remind them of any family history of medical conditions especially things like cancers, heart disease, kidney disease, thyroid problems. and diabetes.

You need to play a huge role in your care and this is a good place to start. Don't forget to review any medications you are on and any over the counter medications and supplements, (including vitamins and herbal), that you are taking.

Slow your life down a notch. I am not saying in your activity, but slow down enough to be thoughtful about safety and preventive health. You don't want your life to be shortened or devastated by a preventable accident or health issue. Making preventive healthcare and safety a priority is the ounce to pay so you don't have to pay the pound of cure, if there is one. Stop… Pause… Think!

Conclusion

I hope this book has helped you become more conscious of the need to be fully engaged in preventive healthcare and safety. We say that the only good accidents and illnesses are the ones we prevent. I can't imagine the number of people who are experiencing severe medical problems and mental anxiety because they know they could have prevented the condition they are in. *"If I had only..."* You fill in the blank. The real sad part is that many of them are sitting where you are right now. You can determine from this day forward, to use every preventive healthcare and safety measure you can to reduce the risk of serious injuries and illnesses.

One more comment for you parents. Parents talk to their children about goals, future plans, college, vocations, relationships, and so many other things. Thousands of children die each year from accidents which could have been prevented so they never did get past high school. Add safety and preventive healthcare to the list of things you can talk to your kids about so you can see all those dreams and plans come true. If I could invent a time machine, I would be a millionaire overnight, because there are so many of us who would love to go back and change something we did or didn't do in the past that is today, causing us painful regrets.

I have been in the medical field for over forty-seven years, and I have seen a lot. My, my, how much sadness, misery, and hurt people live with every day. In many instances, it all could have been prevented. Look at some of the statistics below and then look even more up on the internet. You don't want to increase risk, but rather decrease it. I guarantee you, *An Ounce of Prevention is Worth…More Than You Can Imagine!*

Appendix 1

Preventive Health and Safety Engagement
Statements people should never make... but do!

1. I know I shouldn't cut the grass because it is wet, but I'll be careful.
2. I really don't need anyone steadying the ladder.
3. Someday, we need to get a couple smoke detectors.
4. I am just weed eating a little, I don't need my goggles.
5. I can change this outlet out without turning that breaker off.
6. It saw some lightning, we better hurry to get these last two holes of golf in.
7. I know it says it takes two to lift this box, but I can do it.
8. The step ladder is out in the garage, I'll just use this chair.
9. I keep my safety off when I am hunting so I can shoot quicker.
10. I just going a few miles away, I don't need my seatbelt for that.
11. I get my car inspected at Jo's Tires, they just slap a new sticker on.

12. I know the beach flags are red, but the tide doesn't seem that rough.
13. I forgot my life preserver, but we are not going too far out on the lake.
14. I see the crack in the sidewalk, I'll fix it one of these days.
15. If I get on the ladder, I think I can reach that limb with the chainsaw.
16. I am not texting and driving but I do want to see who it was from.
17. OK little fella, I'll let you sit up front this one time. We are not going far.
18. I should slow down on these windy roads, but I am already late.
19. That baby is really crawling everywhere. We better think about getting the safety outlets someday.
20. I forgot to lock the gate to the pool. No one goes near it though.
21. There would really be no place to hang a fire extinguisher and besides, we have never had even a small fire.
22. The wire is starting to show on that cord. If it gets worse, I'll put some electrician's tape on it.
23. I think if I floor it, I can beat that red light.
24. If I tailgate that slowpoke, maybe he will speed up.
25. I don't need a helmet to ride a bicycle.
26. I am not sure what is at the bottom of the hill, but I am still going to fly down there on my sled.
27. I know that this isn't the beginner's slope, but I'll be careful.
28. I have been shooting for years and I don't wear those silly earplugs.
29. There is my ring, don't touch the garbage disposal switch till I get it out.

30. See who can hold the firecracker the longest before throwing it.
31. OK, see if you can break the record on riding the four-wheeler through the woods.
32. Let's set our bike ramp over that big ditch.
33. That dog looks friendly, I don't think it will bite.
34. We don't have any water for put the campfire out, but it will die out soon.
35. If they sell the toys in a toy store, they have to be safe.
36. All infant car seats are basically the same.
37. I don't need sunscreen; it's supposed to be a little cloudy later.
38. I don't need to stretch, let's go running.
39. It's supposed to warm up a bit. The ice on the porch steps will probably melt.
40. Let's just dive in. The water looks deep enough.

Statistics

Center for Disease Control and **Prevention** Statistics (Unless Designated Otherwise). CDC's main concern isn't reporting statistics but rather **preventing** people from becoming statistics. (That is our goal as well).

1. Over 139,600 people died from lung cancer.
2. 52,000 people died from Colorectal cancer.
3. 45,900 people died from pancreatic cancer.
4. Over 42,000 women died from breast cancer.
5. Over 31,600 men died from prostate cancer.
6. Kidney disease is the 9th leading cause of death in the U.S. An estimated 31 million people in the U.S have kidney disease (about 10% of the adult population) (Kidney Fund.org)
7. 30,000 people died from liver and intrahepatic bile duct cancer.
8. The leading cause of death for children is unintentional injuries.
9. The leading cause of death for children ages 1-4 is drowning.
10. The leading cause of death up to age 44 is unintentional injuries.
11. Over 36,000 people are killed in car accidents each year. (over 2 million injuries).

12. Over 630 children under 12 are killed in car accidents each year. A third of them were not restrained in proper car safety devices. (seat belts, car, and infant seats).
13. Over 2,400 teens are killed in car accidents each year. (Teen Driving Statistics). The numbers are decreasing thankfully but that is still way too many.
14. Over 3,800 people are killed each year in fires. (U.S. Fire Administration) This rate has increased every year since 2014.

The sad part about these statistics is the fact that many of these could have been prevented. Think about all the lives which could be saved if we just realized that, *"An Ounce of Prevention is Worth… More Than You Can Imagine."*

PHASE On!

What is 'P.H.A.S.E. On' All About?

P.H.A.S.E.

Allen Daugherty
Founder (540) 290-4192
www.preventivehealthandsafety.com

Preventive Healthcare and Safety Engagement *A group of caring people, making a difference; one life at a time!*

Our Mission Statement

Our mission is to create public awareness concerning the urgent importance of engaging in Preventive Health and Safety measures to reduce the risk of life-threatening accidents and illnesses.

Our website contains very helpful information. It will constantly be evolving, so keep checking back for new things. We will have videos, interviews, articles and even an affiliate market page to view and purchase various safety and preventive health items.

We are available for speaking engagements for your group no matter what the size. We are not a non-profit organization, but our main goal is to create prevention awareness and not to make a ton of income. The income we generate will be helpful in getting our message out to as many people as we can. We want to save lives and prevent avoidable injuries and illnesses.

How can you help? Starting in the very basic unit, use what you have learned to live a safer and healthier life. Create the same environment in your family as well. Every ounce can help prevent disastrous events from occurring.

Keep your eyes open and help those who you come in contact with. People do so many unsafe things all the time and it's not hard to spot them. Preventive healthcare also carries a much more powerful message when delivered by someone that cares.

Check out our website on ways you can become a *PHASE ON* Member. No money involved, just help us get the message to the masses. Wouldn't you like to get involved in a very simple program that prevents injuries and illnesses? Just think, you could personally save lives. Now that makes life worth living. Join us!

P.H.A.S.E. ON!

www.ingramcontent.com/pod-product-compliance
Lightning Source LLC
Chambersburg PA
CBHW060244030426
42335CB00014B/1587